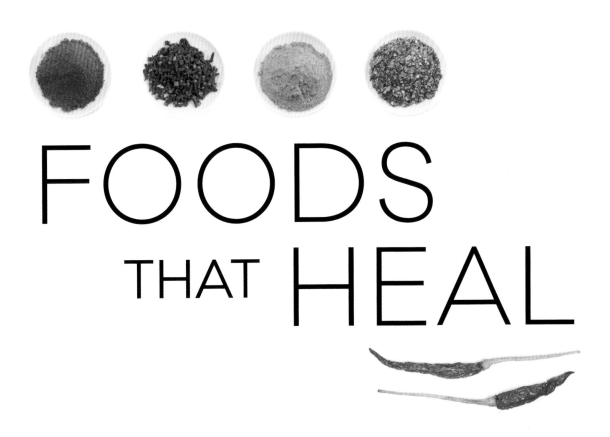

# FOODS
## THAT HEAL

Publications International, Ltd.

**Pictured on the front cover:** Vegetarian Rice Noodles *(page 168)*.

**Pictured on the back cover** *(counterclockwise from top left):* Hot and Sour Soup with Bok Choy and Tofu *(page 52)*, Farro, Chickpea and Spinach Salad *(page 156)*, Blueberry Cherry Blend *(page 40)* and Orange Chicken Stir-Fry over Quinoa *(page 124)*.

ISBN: 978-1-64030-338-6

Manufactured in China.

8 7 6 5 4 3 2 1

# TABLE OF CONTENTS

# FOODS THAT HEAL

There are no magical, miracle foods in the world, but there are plenty of foods that do have great benefits and can help you lead a healthier life. From protecting against heart disease and lowering cholesterol to fighting infection and repairing tissue, certain foods can play a significant role in helping your body heal and function at its best.

The best healing foods are, not surprisingly, minimally processed or whole foods. Foods that are not processed retain more of the balanced combination of nutrients nature gave them—a blend of vitamins, minerals, protein, fiber and other nutrients our bodies need to maintain good health. Whole foods also frequently contain various natural plant substances called phytonutrients that may play important roles in reducing the risk of such ailments as heart disease, high blood pressure, diabetes and cancer.

Ancient civilizations have known about the healing powers of various foods for thousands of years. Scientists today are just beginning to identify substances in these foods and learn more about their potential to heal and protect against disease. Discovering—and taking advantage of—this healing potential may be an important first step in improving and protecting your health. This book, with its clear information and simple recipes, presents a common-sense approach to living a healthy life.

Switching to the right foods can reward you and your family with substantial health benefits and possibly even turn back the clock on aging. As part of a healthy diet, whole foods play a significant role in helping our bodies operate efficiently. Many of these foods provide

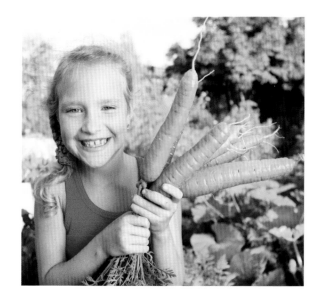

nutrition as well as healing properties, and typically such foods provide multiple healing effects, not just one or two. For example, pineapple was always known to be a good source of vitamin C—important in keeping the immune system strong and prepared to fight infectious diseases—but it also provides a significant amount of manganese, which is essential for energy production and strong bones, and it even contains an enzyme which aids in digestion and reduces inflammation. That's a lot of potential for an often-overlooked fruit!

In this modern world of stores filled with processed foods as well as as medications for every possible ailment, the old adage, "an apple a day keeps the doctor away" might be more true now than ever before. Whether you're fighting an illness, hope to prevent one, or you just want to improve your overall health, you'll find that eating foods that heal the body is a simple recipe for good health—and can provide many surprising and wonderful benefits along the way. The foods profiled in these pages are a great place to start. You'll learn what these foods can do, along with easy and delicious ways to use them.

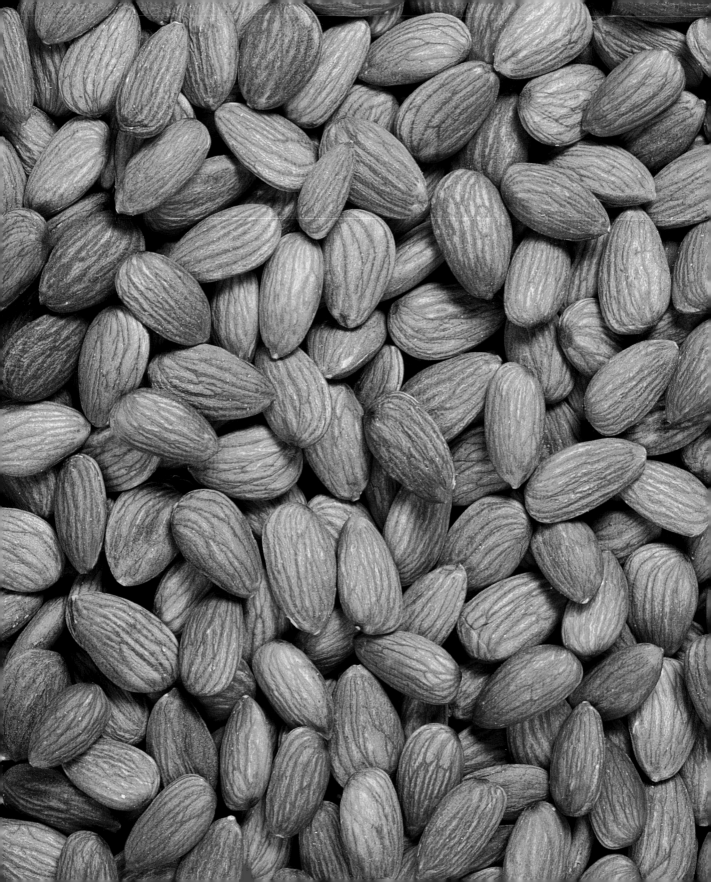

# ALMONDS

These flavorful, nutrient-rich seeds from the fruit of the almond tree pack a powerful nutrient punch in a small package. Versatile almonds are delicious additions to both sweet and savory dishes; they may be used raw, toasted, whole, chopped, or in the forms of almond flour and almond butter.

Ounce for ounce, almonds are one of the most nutrient-dense tree nuts—their combination of protein, fiber and healthy monounsaturated fats provide lasting energy, benefit heart health and overall wellness, and even help reduce cancer risk. Almonds are also a good source of vitamin E and magnesium and provide calcium and B vitamins, as well.

# ALMOND BUTTER

16 ounces lightly salted roasted almonds

2 tablespoons honey

1½ tablespoons safflower oil

**1** Grate almonds in food processor using grating disk. Transfer almonds to large bowl. Remove grating disk; fit processor with metal blade.

**2** Return almonds to food processor; process 2 to 3 minutes or until nuts clump together and form thick paste, scraping side of bowl occasionally.

**3** Add honey and oil; process until desired consistency is reached. Store in airtight container in refrigerator.

*Makes 1½ cups*

# PAPRIKA-SPICED ALMONDS

1 cup whole blanched almonds

¾ teaspoon olive oil

¼ teaspoon coarse salt

¼ teaspoon smoked paprika or paprika

**1** Preheat oven to 375°F. Spread almonds in shallow baking pan.

**2** Bake 8 to 10 minutes or until almonds are lightly browned. Transfer almonds to bowl; cool 5 to 10 minutes.

**3** Drizzle with oil; toss until completely coated. Sprinkle with salt and paprika; toss again.

*Makes about 8 servings*

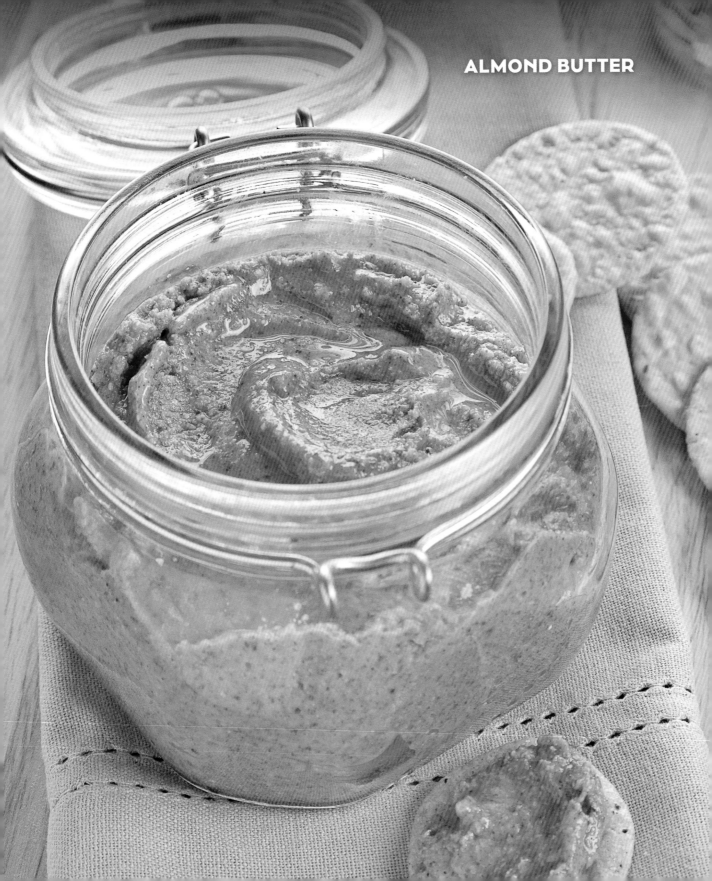

ALMOND BUTTER

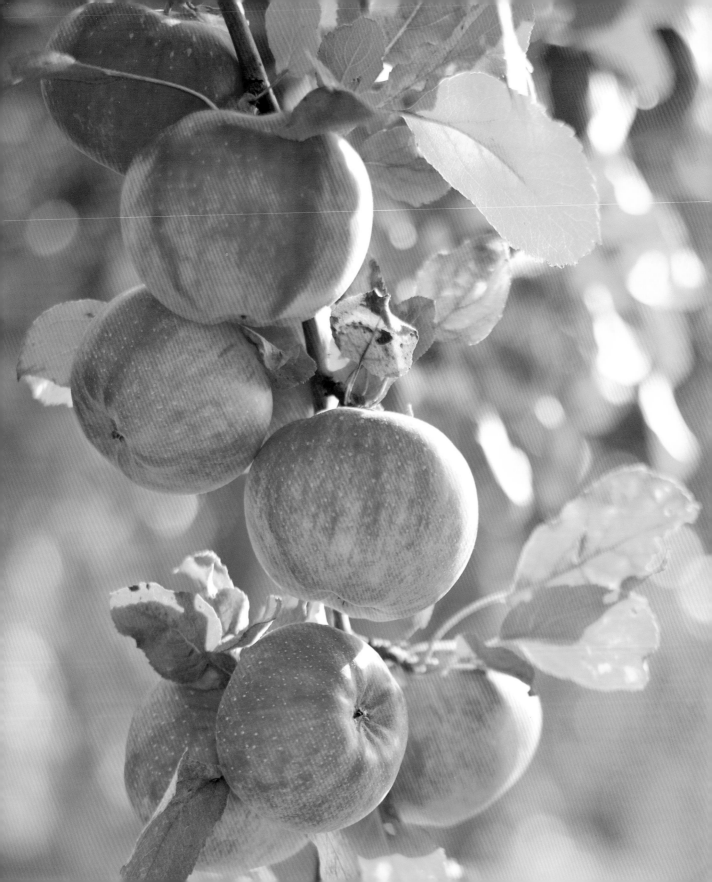

# APPLES

Whether you prefer tart or sweet, extra crunchy or soft and juicy, apples make great low-fat, high-fiber snacks, super desserts and stellar additions to salads and side dishes. There are thousands of apple varieties to choose from, so don't limit yourself to one or two.

The soluble fiber in apples may help keep blood cholesterol levels in check, while apples also provide vitamin C, an antioxidant that may help prevent heart disease and some cancers. Regularly snacking on apples may even help maintain a healthy smile on your face by stimulating your gums and keeping your breath fresh.

# WHEAT BERRY APPLE SALAD

1 **cup uncooked wheat berries (whole wheat kernels)**

½ **teaspoon salt**

2 **apples (1 red and 1 green)**

1 **stalk celery, chopped**

½ **cup dried cranberries**

⅓ **cup chopped walnuts**

**Grated peel and juice of 1 medium orange**

2 **tablespoons rice wine vinegar**

1½ **tablespoons chopped fresh mint**

**Lettuce leaves (optional)**

**1** Combine wheat berries and salt in large saucepan; cover with 1 inch of water.* Bring to a boil over high heat. Stir wheat berries. Reduce heat to low; cover and cook 45 minutes to 1 hour or until wheat berries are tender but chewy, stirring occasionally. (Add additional water if wheat berries become dry during cooking.) Drain and let cool. (Refrigerate up to 4 days if not using immediately.)

**2** Cut apples into bite-size pieces. Combine wheat berries, apples, celery, cranberries, walnuts, orange peel, orange juice, vinegar and mint in large bowl; toss to coat. Cover and refrigerate at least 1 hour to allow flavors to blend.

**3** Serve salad on lettuce leaves, if desired.

*To cut cooking time by 20 to 30 minutes, wheat berries may be soaked in water overnight. Drain and cover with 1 inch fresh water before cooking.*

***Makes about 6 cups***

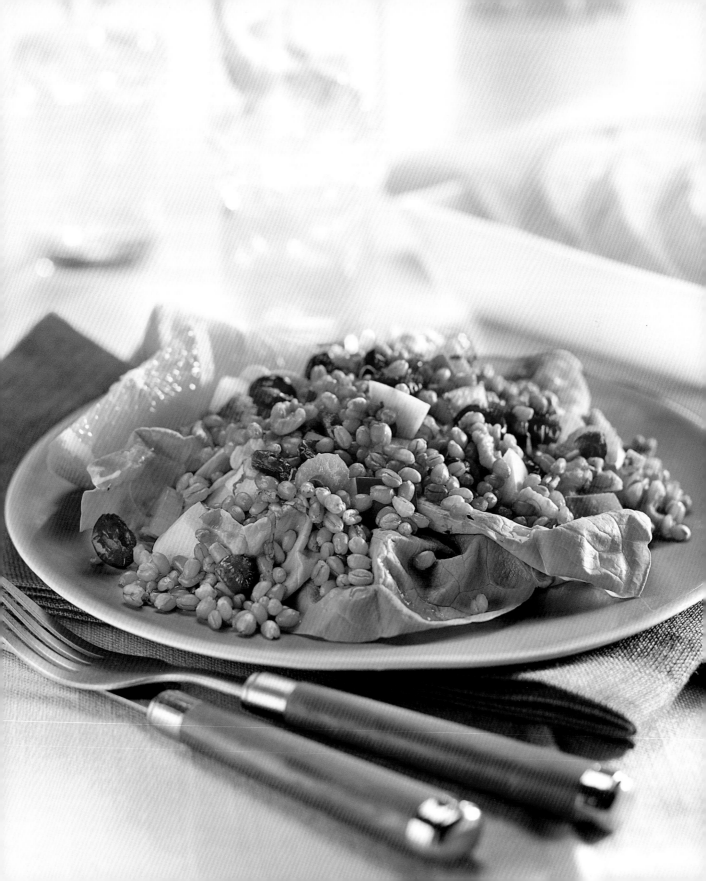

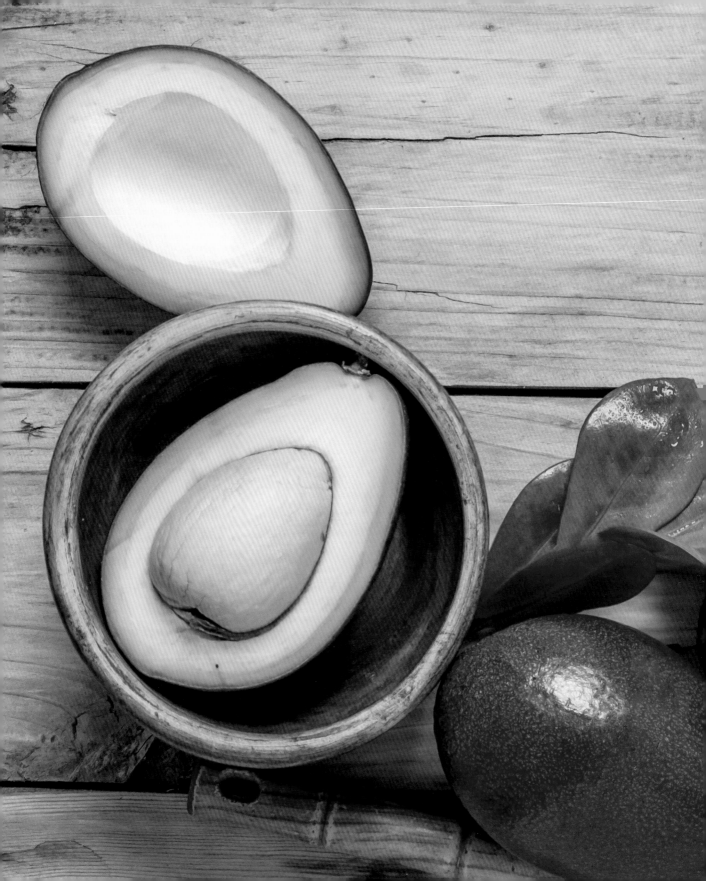

# AVOCADO

This deliciously rich, smooth-textured fruit is often mistaken for a vegetable—and its buttery flavor is an excellent addition to vegetable, meat, salad and pasta dishes. In its simplest form, it is widely enjoyed mashed, seasoned and served as guacamole or spread on toast.

Avocados are rich in monounsaturated fat, a type of fat that can help lower LDL "bad" cholesterol, especially when it replaces saturated fat. Avocados contain more potassium than bananas, and some studies have shown that a high potassium intake is linked to reduced blood pressure. Avocados are a good source of fiber, minerals, folate, which is crucial for cell repair, and B vitamins, which help fight off disease and infection. Avocados also contain lutein, an antioxidant that helps maintain healthy eyes and skin.

# TOMATO, AVOCADO AND CUCUMBER SALAD

1½ tablespoons extra virgin
   olive oil

1 tablespoon balsamic vinegar

1 clove garlic, minced

¼ teaspoon salt

¼ teaspoon black pepper

2 cups diced seeded plum
   tomatoes

1 small ripe avocado, cut
   into ½-inch pieces

½ cup chopped cucumber

⅓ cup crumbled feta cheese

4 large red leaf lettuce leaves

Chopped fresh basil (optional)

**1** Whisk oil, vinegar, garlic, salt and pepper in medium bowl. Add tomatoes and avocado; toss gently to coat. Stir in cucumber and cheese.

**2** Arrange one lettuce leaf on each serving plate. Spoon salad evenly onto lettuce leaves. Top with basil, if desired.

*Makes 4 servings*

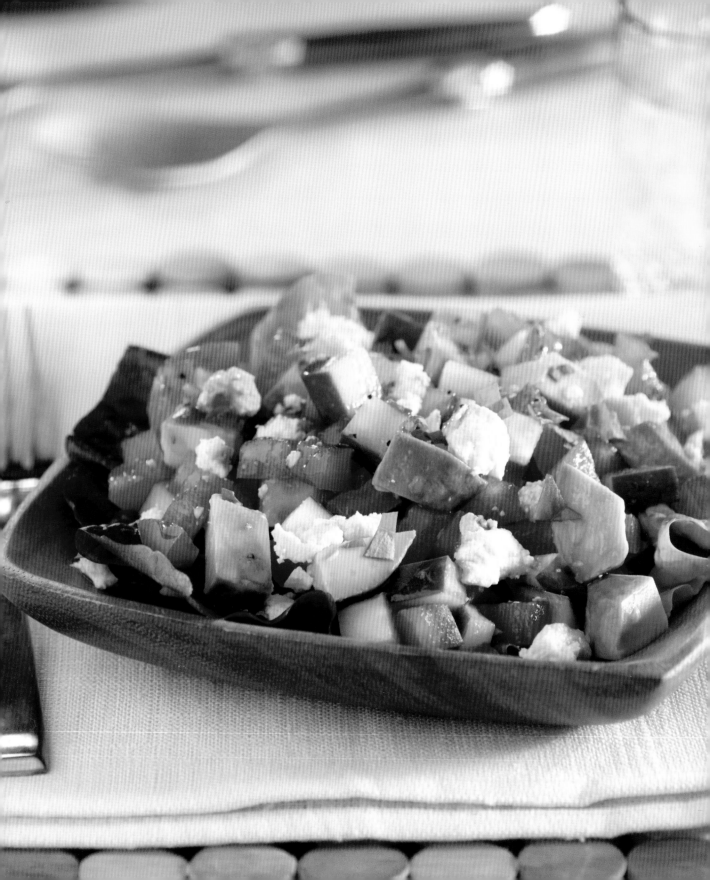

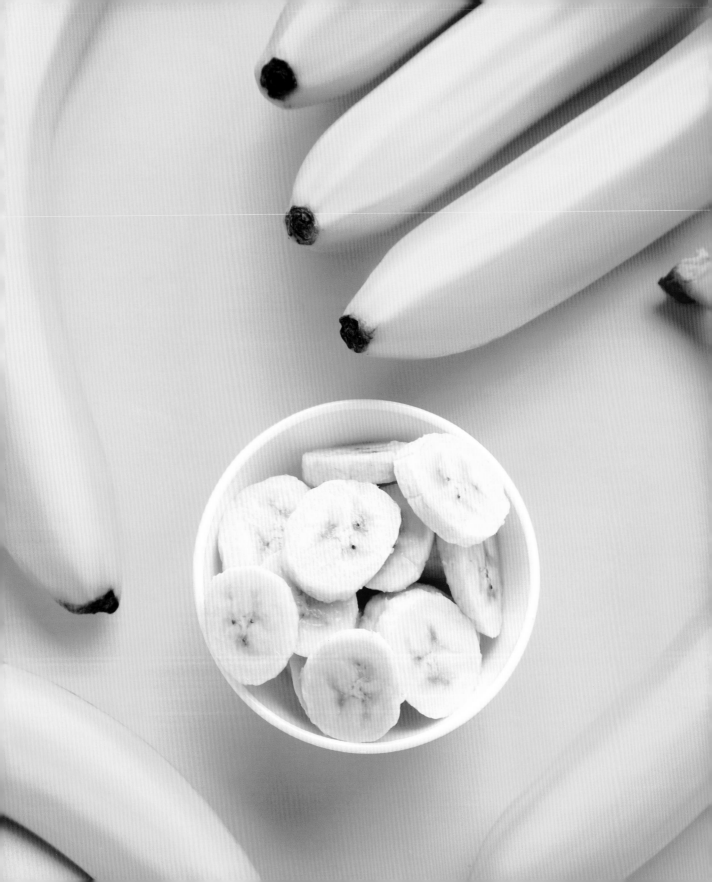

# BANANAS

Bananas are one of the most popular fruits in the United States—they're the perfect portable snack, and their tropical sweetness adds a bit of sunshine any time of day.

Bananas are fat free and high in fiber, which makes them filling and also helps keep your digestive tract functioning well. Bananas are loaded with potassium, and research shows that getting enough potassium—and cutting back on sodium—may be important for bringing high blood pressure under control. Plus, bananas supply vitamin C, which helps your immune system perform at its peak.

# BLUEBERRY BANANA OATMEAL SMOOTHIE

1 **cup milk**

1 **banana**

½ **cup frozen blueberries**

½ **cup plain yogurt**

¼ **cup quick oats**

Combine milk, banana and blueberries in blender; blend until smooth. Add yogurt and oats; blend until smooth.

*Makes 2 servings*

# PEANUT BUTTER BANANA BLEND

½ **cup milk**

½ **cup plain yogurt**

1 **frozen banana**

1 **tablespoon all-natural unsweetened peanut butter**

Combine milk, yogurt, banana and peanut butter in blender; blend until smooth.

*Makes 2 servings*

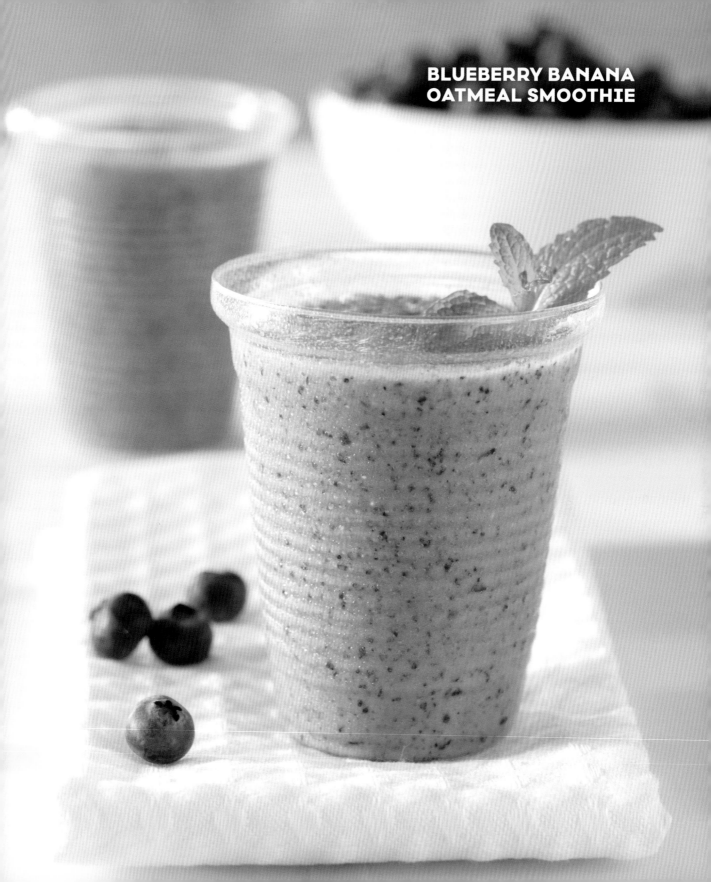

BLUEBERRY BANANA
OATMEAL SMOOTHIE

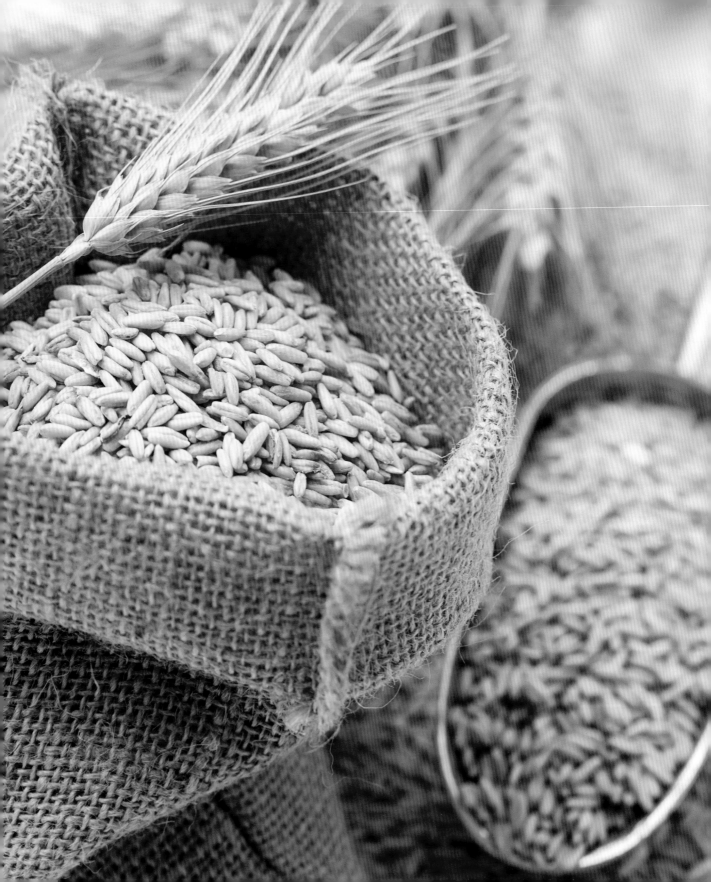

# BARLEY

This versatile, fiber-rich grain is typically used in soups, stews and casseroles; its nutty flavor and slightly chewy texture also make barley a satisfying change from rice.

Barley contains beta-glucan, the same cholesterol-lowering soluble fiber found in oat bran and dried beans. Barley is rich in insoluble fiber as well, absorbing water so it adds bulk and speeds intestinal contents through your body, which may reduce your risk for colorectal cancers. Insoluble fiber may also help keep digestive disorders like constipation at bay. And barley helps control blood sugar levels and improve insulin response, reducing the risk of type 2 diabetes.

# BARLEY AND VEGETABLE RISOTTO

4½ cups vegetable or chicken
   broth

2 teaspoons olive oil

1 small onion, diced

8 ounces sliced mushrooms

¾ cup uncooked pearl barley

1 large red bell pepper, diced

2 cups packed baby spinach

¼ cup grated Parmesan cheese

¼ teaspoon black pepper

**1** Bring broth to a boil in medium saucepan over high heat; keep warm over low heat.

**2** Meanwhile, heat oil in large saucepan over medium heat. Add onion; cook and stir 4 minutes. Add mushrooms; cook over medium-high heat 5 minutes or until mushrooms begin to brown and liquid evaporates, stirring frequently.

**3** Add barley; cook 1 minute. Add broth, ¼ cup at a time, stirring constantly until broth is almost absorbed before adding next ¼ cup.

**4** After 20 minutes of cooking, stir in bell pepper. Continue adding broth, ¼ cup at a time, until barley is tender (about 30 minutes total). Stir in spinach; cook and stir 1 minute or just until spinach is wilted. Stir in cheese and black pepper.

*Makes 4 to 6 servings*

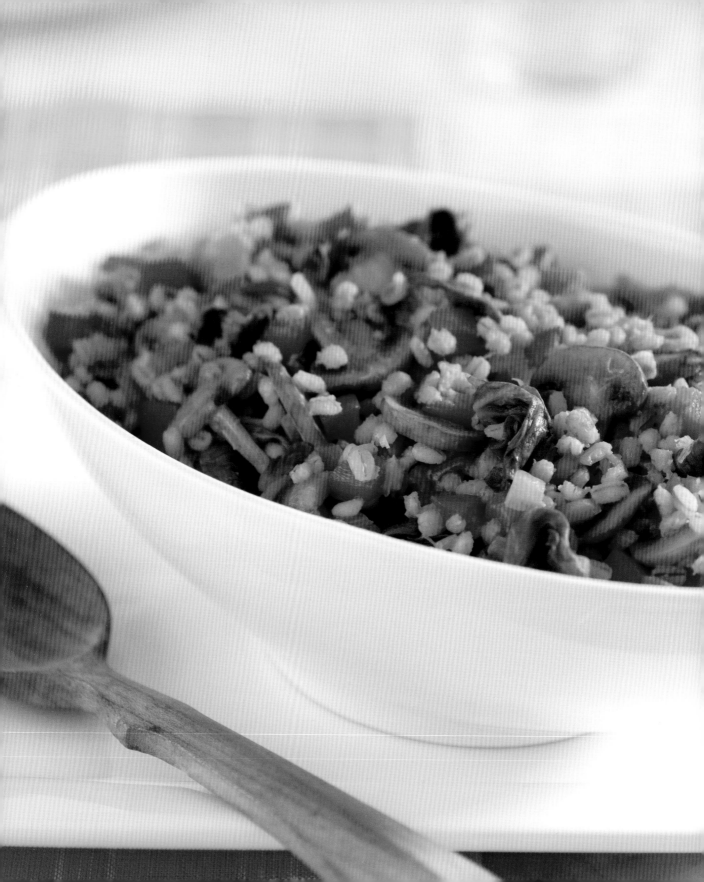

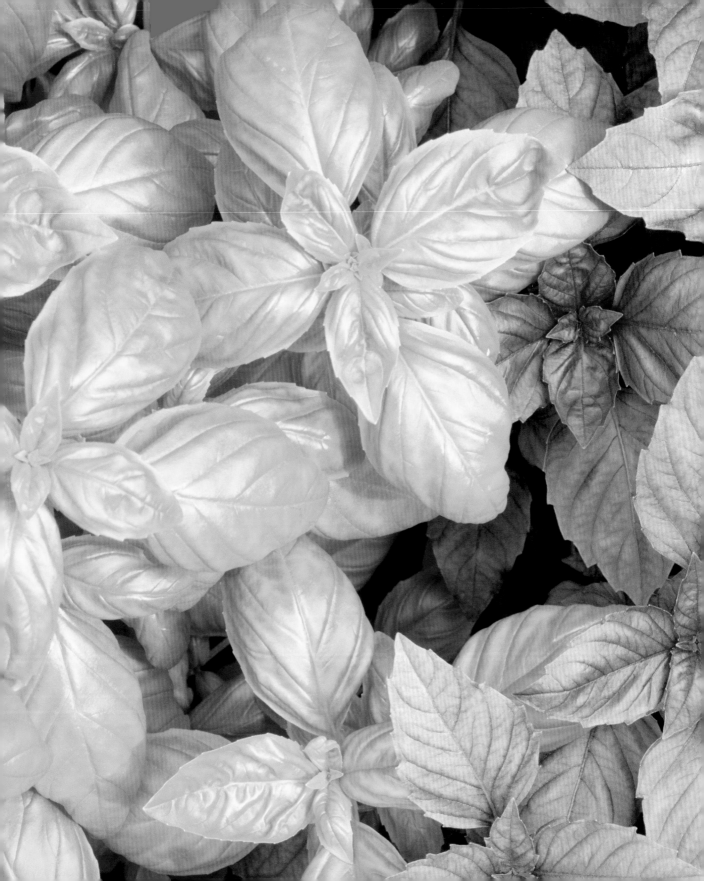

# BASIL

This popular aromatic herb, a member of the mint family, contains essential oils that have been shown to lower blood glucose, trigyceride and cholesterol levels. Fresh basil contains flavonoids and beta-carotene, powerful antioxidants that protect the body's cells from damage which can lead to disease. And basil is a rich source of magnesium, which promotes cardiovascular health by prompting muscles and blood vessels to relax, improving blood flow throughout the body.

# BAKED FISH
## WITH THAI PESTO

1 to 2 jalapeño peppers,*
   coarsely chopped

1 lemon

4 green onions, thinly sliced

2 tablespoons chopped
   fresh ginger

3 cloves garlic, minced

1½ cups lightly packed fresh
   basil leaves

1 cup lightly packed fresh
   cilantro leaves

¼ cup lightly packed fresh
   mint leaves

¼ cup roasted peanuts
   (salted or unsalted)

2 tablespoons sweetened
   shredded coconut

½ teaspoon sugar

½ cup peanut oil

2 pounds boneless fish fillets
   (such as salmon, halibut,
   cod or orange roughy)

   Lemon and cucumber slices

*Jalapeño peppers can sting and
irritate the skin, so wear rubber
gloves when handling peppers
and do not touch your eyes.*

1 Place jalapeño peppers in blender or
   food processor.

2 Grate peel of lemon. Juice lemon to
   measure 2 tablespoons. Add peel and
   juice to blender.

3 Add green onions, ginger, garlic, basil,
   cilantro, mint, peanuts, coconut and sugar
   to blender; blend until finely chopped.
   With motor running, slowly pour in oil;
   blend until almost smooth.

4 Preheat oven to 375°F. Rinse fish and
   pat dry with paper towels. Place on
   lightly oiled baking sheet. Spread solid
   thin layer of pesto over each fillet.

5 Bake 10 minutes or until fish begins to
   flake when tested with fork and is just
   opaque in center. Garnish with lemon
   and cucumber.

*Makes 4 to 6 servings*

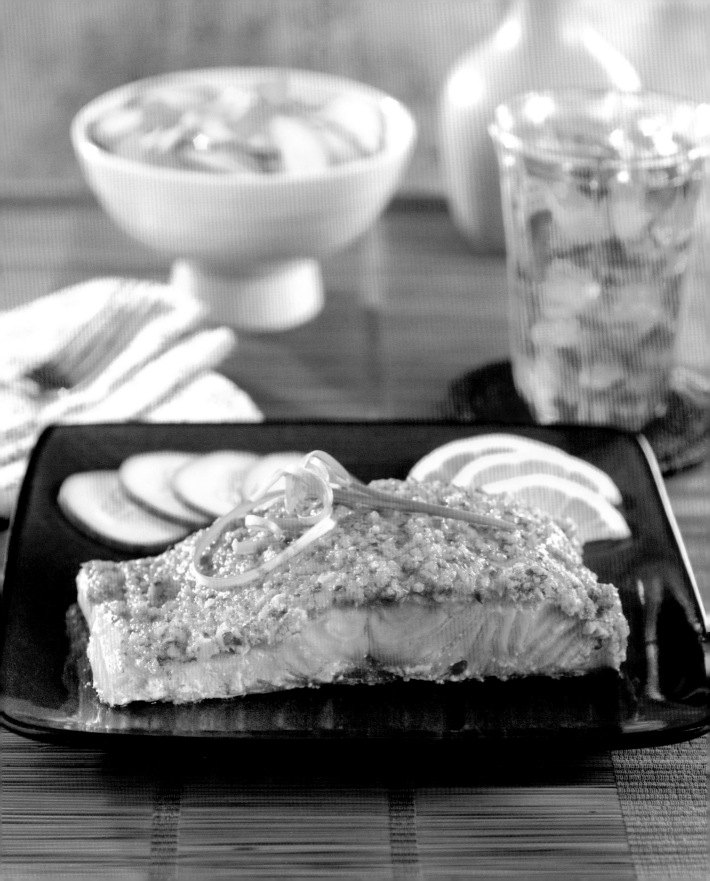

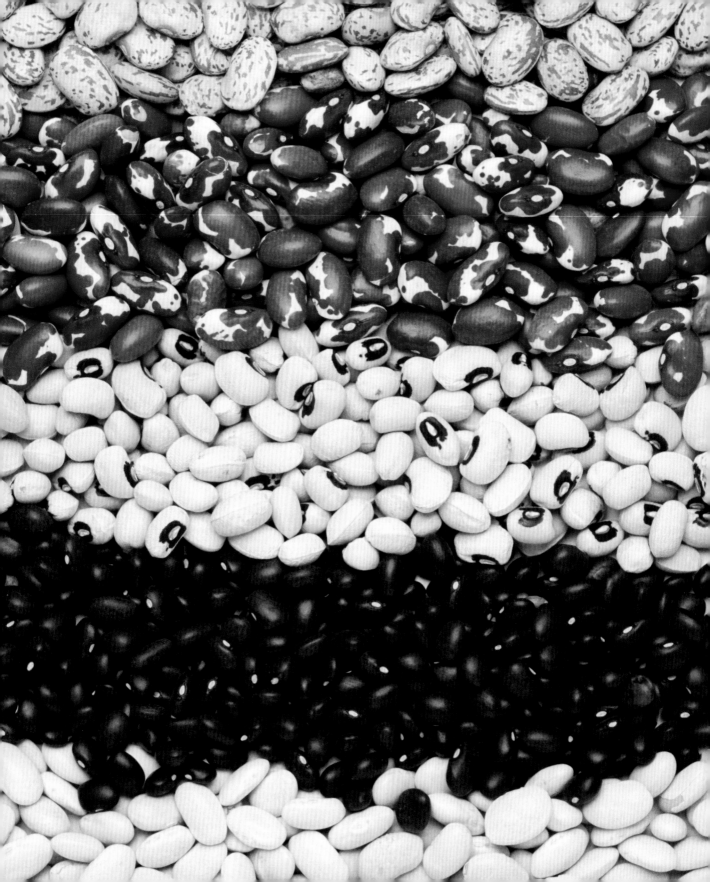

# BEANS

High in protein, low in fat and containing more fiber than most whole grains, beans have been a food staple in many cultures for thousands of years. It's hard to beat these versatile legumes as a healthy and economical source of essential nutrients.

According to research, diets that include beans are associated with lower risks of heart disease and some cancers. The soluble fiber in beans slows digestion and blunts the rise of blood sugar after meals. Beans also provide significant amounts of folate, manganese, magnesium, copper, iron and potassium—nutrients many of us get too little of. And their protein and iron make beans all but essential for people who don't eat meat.

# CHUNKY BLACK BEAN
## AND SWEET POTATO CHILI

2 teaspoons olive oil

1 cup chopped sweet onion

2 red or green bell peppers
   or 1 of each, cut into
   ½-inch pieces

4 cloves garlic, minced

1 teaspoon chili powder

1 can (about 14 ounces) fire-
   roasted diced tomatoes

1 small sweet potato (8 ounces),
   peeled and cut into ½-inch
   pieces (1½ cups)

1 tablespoon minced canned
   chipotle peppers in adobo
   sauce

1 can (about 15 ounces) black
   beans, rinsed and drained

½ cup chopped fresh cilantro
   (optional)

1 Heat oil in large saucepan over medium heat. Add onion; cook and stir 5 minutes. Add bell peppers, garlic and chili powder; cook and stir 2 minutes.

2 Stir in tomatoes, sweet potato and chipotle peppers; bring to a boil. Reduce heat to medium-low; cover and cook 15 minutes.

3 Stir in black beans; cover and cook 8 to 10 minutes or until vegetables are tender. (Chili will be thick; thin with water as desired.)

4 Top with cilantro, if desired.

*Makes 4 servings*

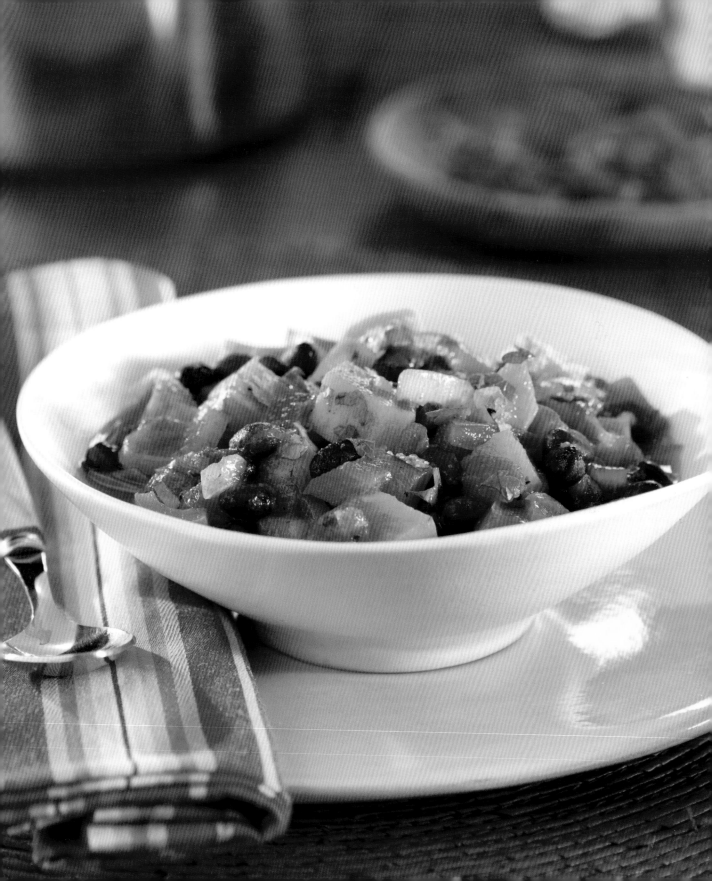

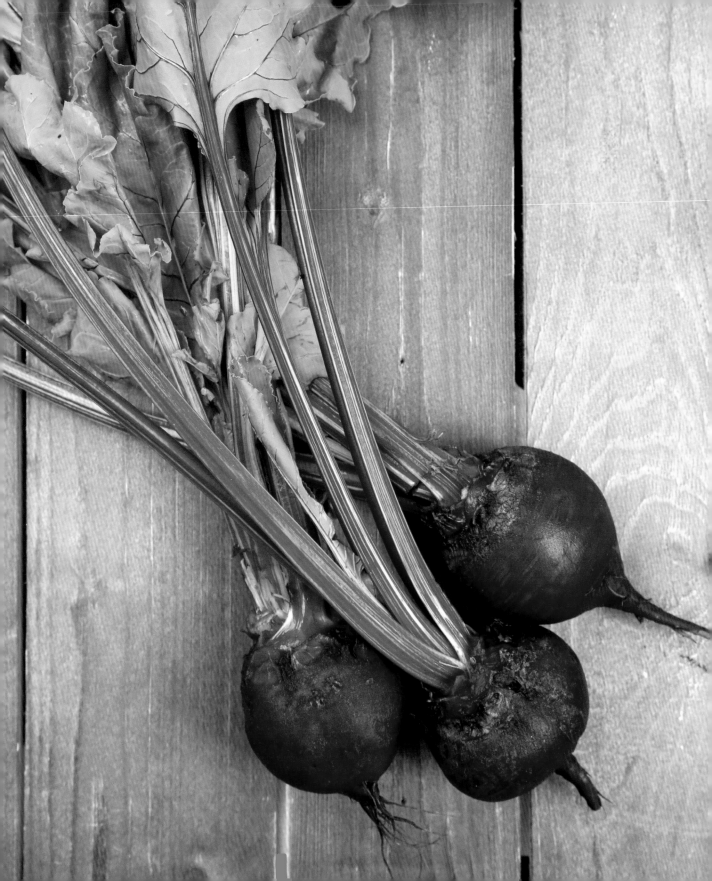

# BEETS

Known for their deep colors and earthy flavor, beets—and their greens—offer incredible nutritional value. Beets contain a wealth of fiber, half soluble and half insoluble. Their rich nutrient and fiber loads and low carbohydrate and calorie counts make them effective tools for blood sugar control.

Beets are particularly rich in folate, fiber and potassium while their greens are full of calcium, iron, beta-carotene and vitamin C. Beets are also high in phytonutrients, which may help lower cholesterol levels.

# CIDER VINAIGRETTE-GLAZED BEETS

6 **medium beets**

2 **tablespoons olive oil**

1 **tablespoon cider vinegar**

½ **teaspoon prepared horseradish**

½ **teaspoon Dijon mustard**

¼ **teaspoon packed brown sugar**

⅓ **cup crumbled blue cheese (optional)**

**1** Cut tops off beets, leaving at least 1 inch of stems. Scrub beets under cold running water with soft vegetable brush, being careful not to break skins.

**2** Place beets in large saucepan; add water to cover. Bring to a boil over high heat. Reduce heat to low; simmer 30 minutes or just until beets are barely firm when pierced with fork. Transfer to plate to cool slightly.

**3** Meanwhile, whisk oil, vinegar, horseradish, mustard and brown sugar in medium bowl until well blended.

**4** When beets are cool enough to handle, peel off skins and trim off root end. Cut beets into halves, then into wedges. Add warm beets to vinaigrette; toss gently to coat. Sprinkle with cheese, if desired. Serve warm or at room temperature.

*Makes 6 servings*

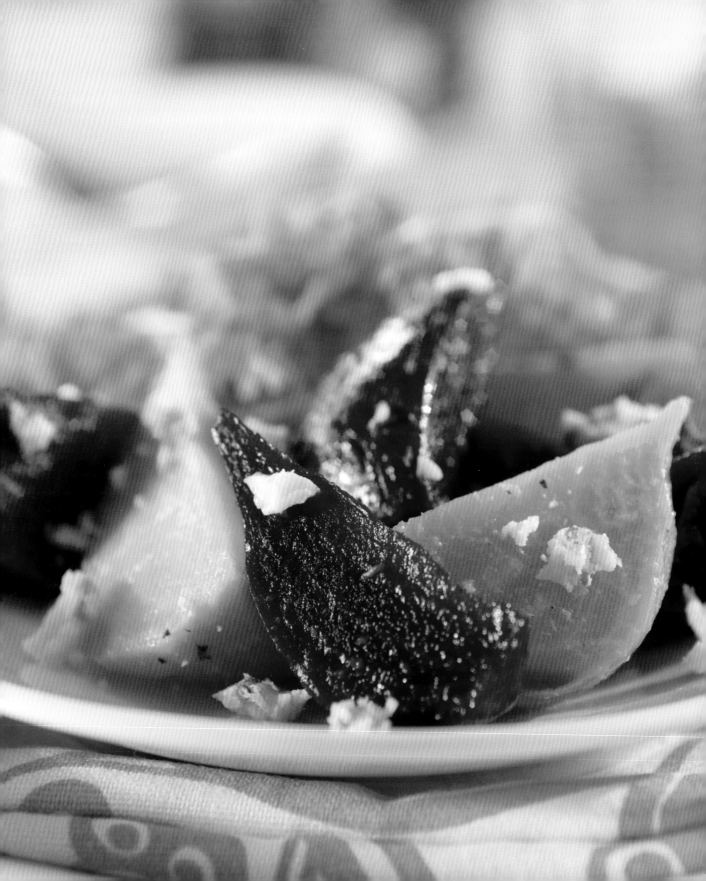

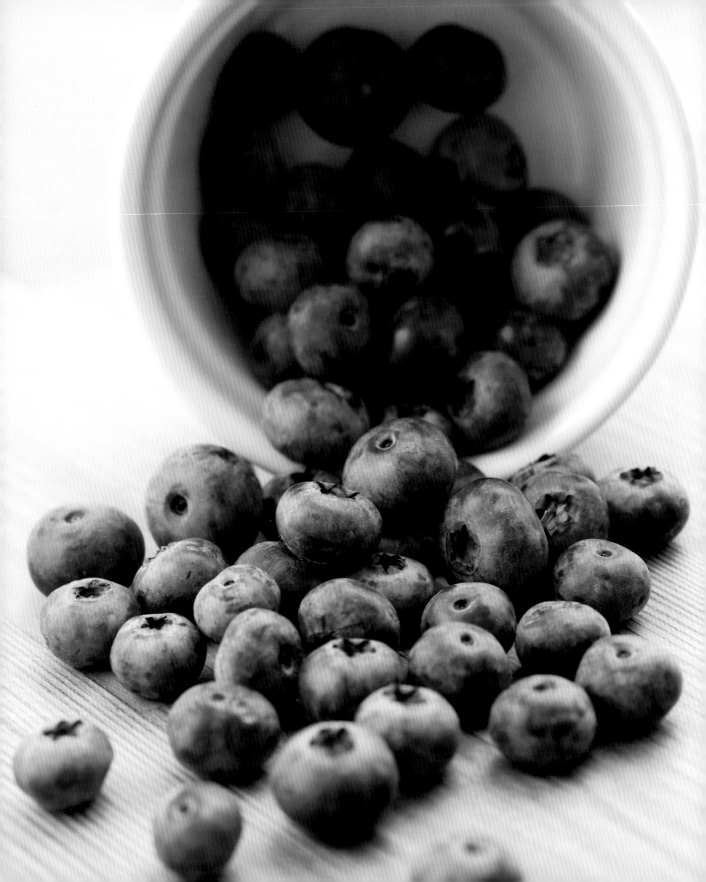

# BLUEBERRIES

Powerfully nutritious, blueberries are antioxidant superstars, ranking second among top antioxidant-rich foods. These popular berries add color and flavor to everything from pancakes to salads to blueberry pie.

Research shows the antioxidants in blueberries may protect brain cells and help reverse age-related memory loss. And as part of a healthy diet, eating blueberries may help reduce several key risk factors for cardiovascular disease and diabetes, such as high blood cholesterol, high blood sugar and accumulation of belly fat. In addition, blueberries contain anthocyanins, the phytonutrients that give them their distinctive blue-purple color and may help prevent heart disease and cancer. Blueberries also provide both iron and vitamin C, an especially beneficial combination because vitamin C enables the body to better absorb the iron in plant foods. And similar to cranberries, blueberries can help treat and prevent urinary tract infections.

# BLUEBERRY CHERRY BLEND

¾  **cup water**

¾  **cup frozen blueberries**

¾  **cup frozen dark sweet cherries**

½  **avocado**

1  **tablespoon lemon juice**

1  **teaspoon ground flaxseed**

Combine water, blueberries, cherries, avocado, lemon juice and flaxseed in blender; blend until smooth.

*Makes 2 servings*

# PURPLE PICK-ME-UP

¼  **cup water**

1  **navel orange, peeled and seeded**

1  **cup frozen blueberries**

4  **Medjool dates, pitted**

Combine water, orange, blueberries and dates in blender; blend until smooth.

*Makes 2 servings*

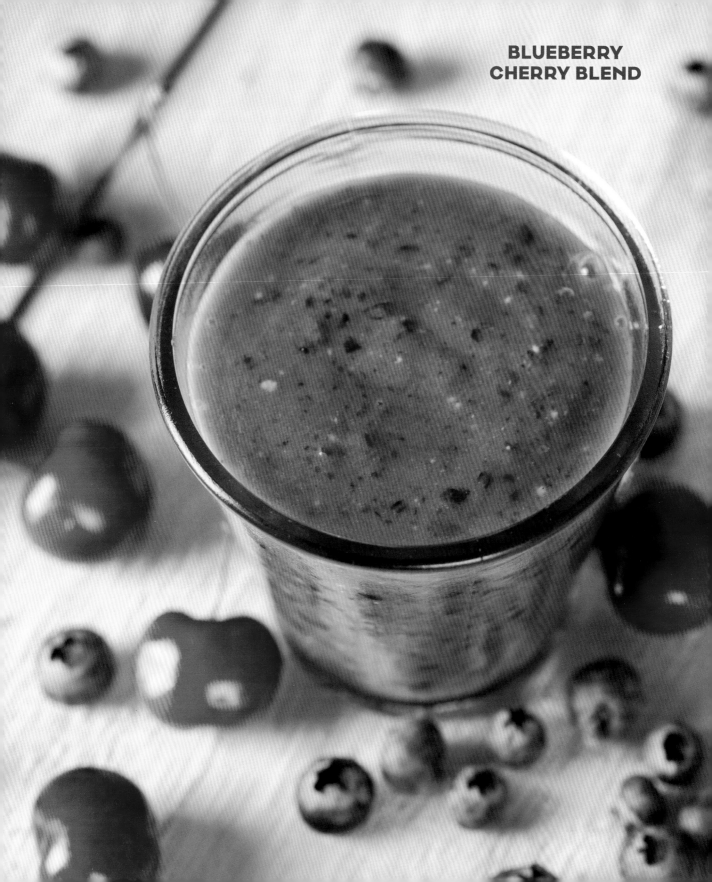

**BLUEBERRY CHERRY BLEND**

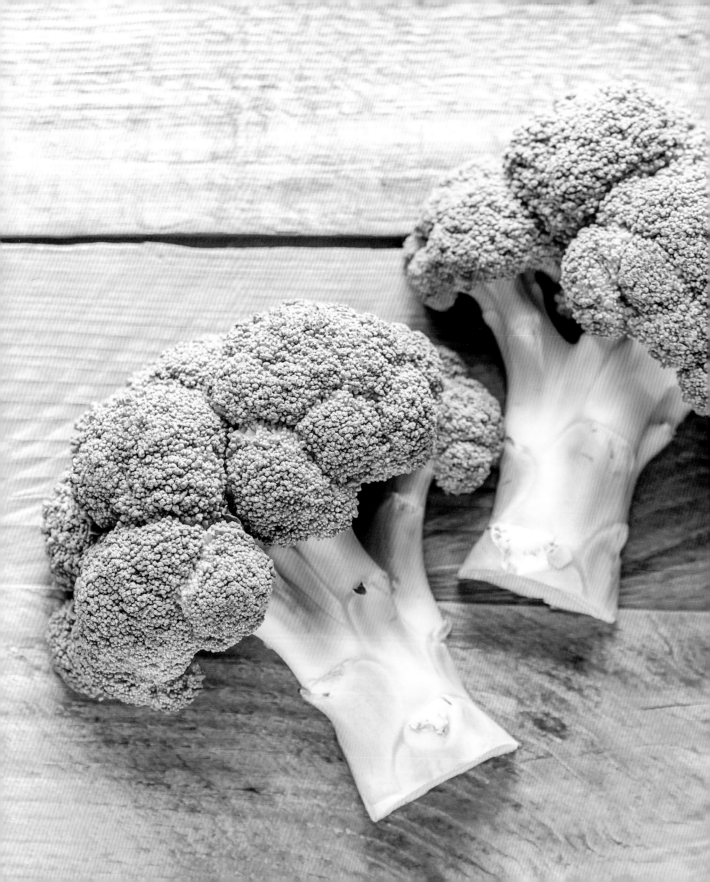

# BROCCOLI

Broccoli provides a hefty dose of disease-fighting nutrients, which is particularly impressive for a vegetable so low in sugars and carbohydrates.

This cruciferous vegetable is packed with vitamin C, vitamin A (mostly as the antioxidant beta-carotene), folate and calcium, a nutrient roster that is especially beneficial for women, since adequate folate intake before and during pregnancy helps prevent neural-tube birth defects. And getting enough calcium can help prevent osteoporosis. Broccoli is rich in various phytonutrients that serve as powerful cancer fighters, helping to inhibit tumor growth and boost the action of protective enzymes. Broccoli is also a rich source of both soluble fiber (good for heart health) and insoluble fiber (helps to keep your digestive tract intact).

# BROCCOLI ITALIAN STYLE

1½  pounds fresh broccoli

1¼  teaspoons salt, divided

2  tablespoons lemon juice

2  tablespoons extra virgin
   olive oil

1  tablespoon chopped fresh
   Italian parsley

1  clove garlic, minced

⅛  teaspoon black pepper

**1** Trim broccoli, discarding tough stems. Cut broccoli into florets with 2-inch stems. Peel remaining stems; cut into ½-inch slices.

**2** Bring 1 quart water and 1 teaspoon salt to a boil in large saucepan over medium-high heat. Add broccoli; return to a boil. Cook 3 to 5 minutes or until tender. Drain broccoli; transfer to serving dish.

**3** Whisk lemon juice, oil, parsley, garlic, remaining ¼ teaspoon salt and pepper in small bowl until well blended. Pour over broccoli; toss to coat. Cover and let stand 1 hour before serving to allow flavors to blend. Serve at room temperature.

*Makes 4 servings*

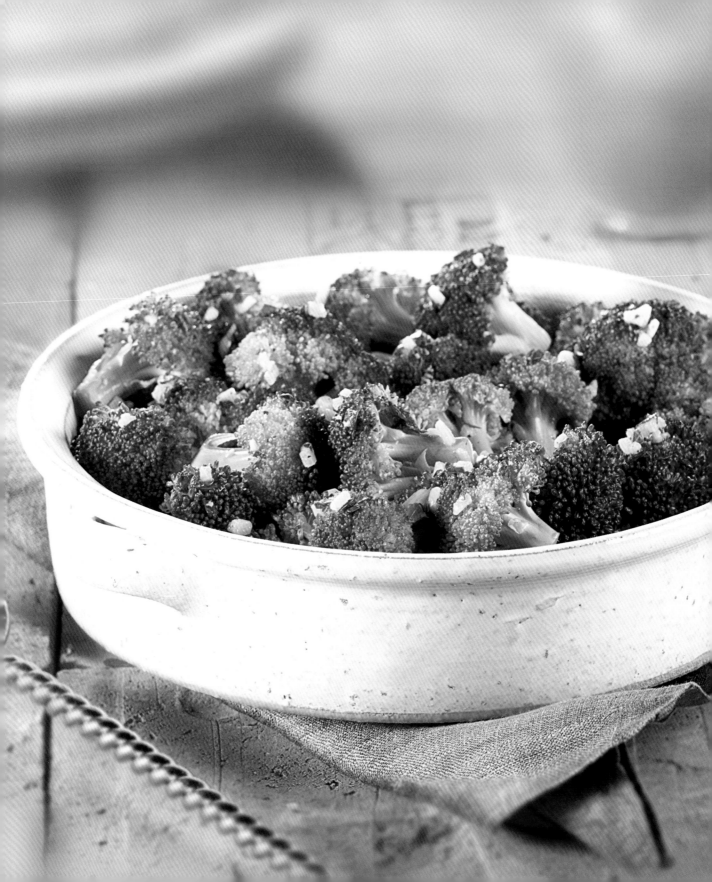

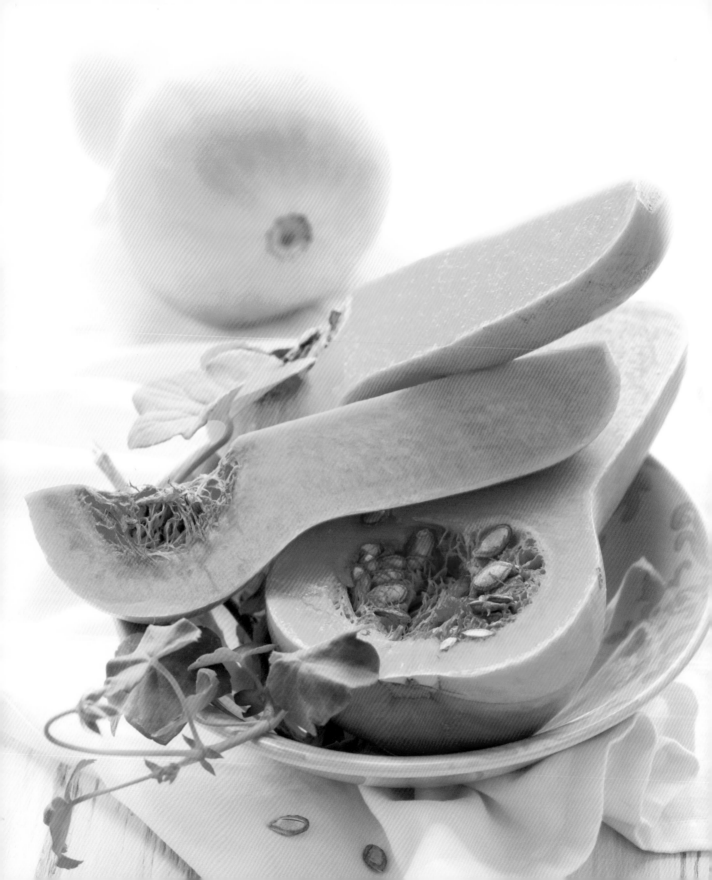

# BUTTERNUT SQUASH

This sweet, satisfying and fiber-rich winter squash takes a bit of work to get beyond the tough skin, but it makes an excellent addition to any meal.

The fiber in butternut squash provides a feeling of fullness and slows the rise in blood sugar levels after a meal. Beta-carotene, the antioxidant form of vitamin A, gives butternut squash its deep orange-yellow color. This essential vitamin helps maintain eye health, promotes healthy skin, and protects the body's cells from harm caused by exposure to tobacco, sunlight, radiation and other potentially cancer-causing substances. It's also a good source of vitamin C, which is essential for a healthy immune system.

# SPICY SQUASH AND CHICKEN SOUP

1 tablespoon olive oil

1 small onion, finely chopped

1 stalk celery, finely chopped

2 cups cubed butternut squash (about 1 small)

2 cups chicken broth

1 can (about 14 ounces) diced tomatoes with green chiles

1 cup chopped cooked chicken

½ teaspoon salt

½ teaspoon ground ginger

⅛ teaspoon ground cumin

⅛ teaspoon black pepper

2 teaspoons lime juice

Fresh parsley or cilantro sprigs (optional)

**1** Heat oil in large saucepan over medium heat. Add onion and celery; cook and stir 5 minutes or until vegetables are tender.

**2** Stir in squash, broth, tomatoes, chicken, salt, ginger, cumin and pepper; cover and cook over low heat 30 minutes or until squash is tender.

**3** Stir in lime juice; garnish with parsley.

***Makes 4 servings***

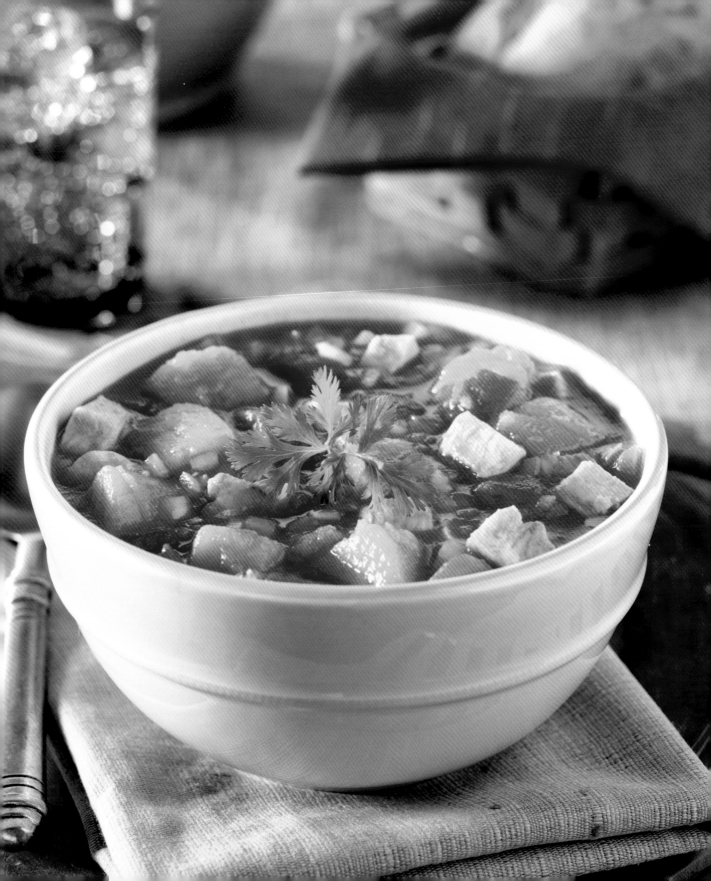

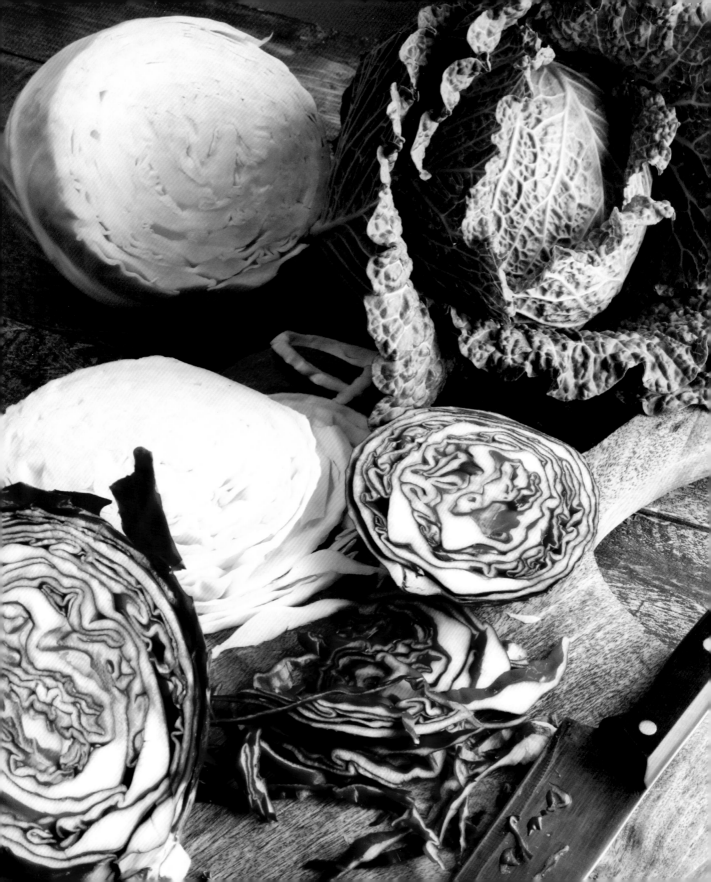

# CABBAGE

Available in hundreds of varieties, cabbage contains a wealth of important nutrients. It contains both soluble and insoluble fiber and a significant amount of vitamin K, which helps maintain bone strength and plays an important role in proper blood clotting.

Researchers have found that eating leafy green vegetables, such as cabbage, may reduce the risk of developing type 2 diabetes. For those who already have diabetes, cabbage offers fiber to help slow blood sugar's rise during a meal. Bok choy cabbage is an important nondairy source of calcium, which helps to prevent osteoporosis and control blood pressure. Savoy and bok choy cabbages provide beta-carotene, which reduces risks of heart disease and cancer.

# HOT AND SOUR SOUP WITH BOK CHOY AND TOFU

1 tablespoon dark sesame oil

4 ounces shiitake mushrooms, stems finely chopped, caps thinly sliced

2 cloves garlic, minced

2 cups mushroom or vegetable broth

1 cup plus 2 tablespoons cold water, divided

2 tablespoons reduced-sodium soy sauce

1½ tablespoons rice or white wine vinegar

¼ teaspoon red pepper flakes

1½ tablespoons cornstarch

2 cups coarsely chopped bok choy leaves or napa cabbage

10 ounces silken extra firm tofu, well drained, cut into ½-inch cubes

1 green onion, thinly sliced

**1** Heat oil in large saucepan over medium heat. Add mushrooms and garlic; cook and stir 3 minutes. Add broth, 1 cup water, soy sauce, vinegar and red pepper flakes; bring to a boil. Reduce heat to medium-low; simmer 5 minutes.

**2** Whisk remaining 2 tablespoons water into cornstarch in small bowl until smooth. Stir into soup; cook 2 minutes or until thickened.

**3** Stir in bok choy; cook 2 to 3 minutes or until wilted. Stir in tofu; cook until heated through. Sprinkle with green onion.

*Makes 4 servings*

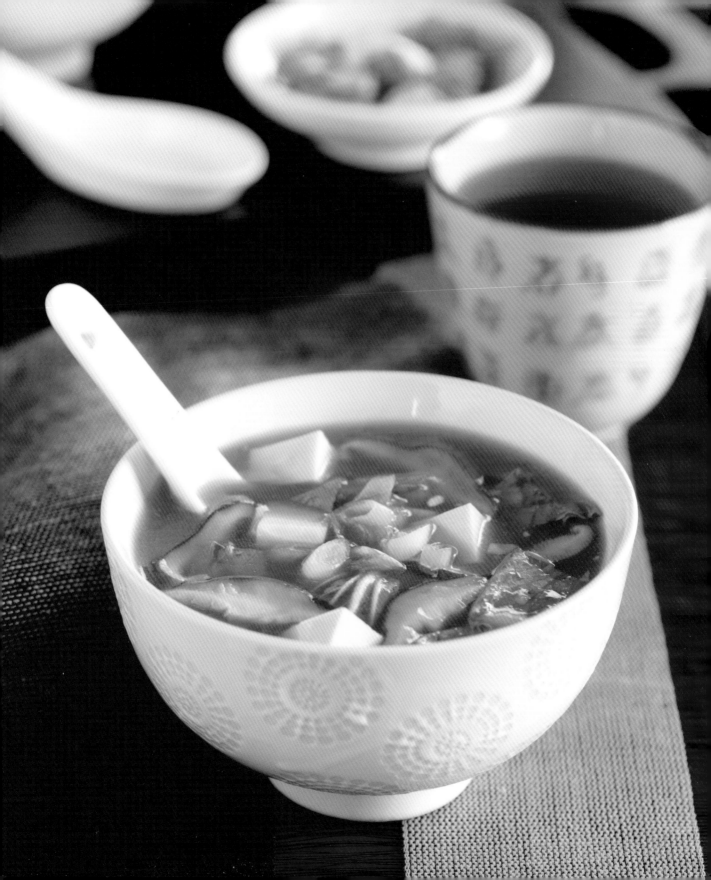

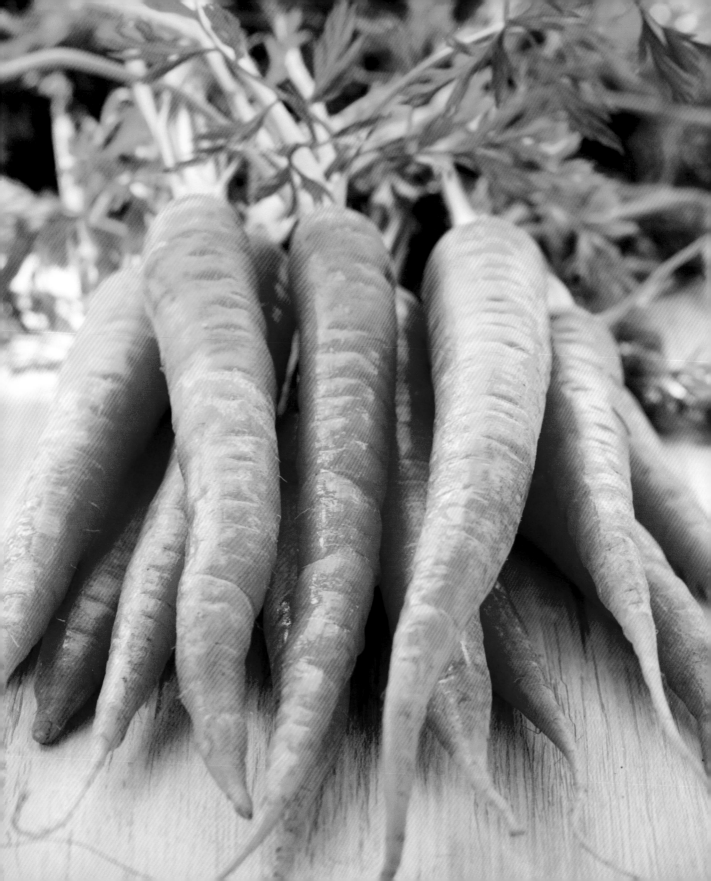

# CARROTS

Carrots may be considered an unexciting or ordinary vegetable, but they are anything but ordinary when it comes to nutrition.

Sweet, crunchy carrots are a super food, containing an enormous amount of beta-carotene. This type of vitamin A helps protect eyesight, including night vision, and helps prevent macular degeneration and cataracts, two leading causes of blindness in people 55 and older. That same vitamin A also helps to keep the skin healthy and supple and the body shielded from infections of all kinds. It's a potent cancer fighter, too. And the soluble fiber helps lower blood cholesterol levels and fight hunger.

# ROASTED PARSNIPS, CARROTS AND RED ONION

2 carrots (9 ounces), cut into 2-inch-long pieces

2 parsnips (9 ounces), cut into 2-inch-long pieces

¾ cup vertically sliced red onion (¼-inch slices)

2 tablespoons extra virgin olive oil

1 tablespoon balsamic vinegar

¼ teaspoon salt

⅛ teaspoon black pepper

1 Preheat oven to 425°F. Line large baking sheet with foil or spray with nonstick cooking spray.

2 Combine carrots, parsnips, onion, oil, vinegar, salt and pepper in large bowl; toss to coat. Spread in single layer on prepared baking sheet.

3 Roast 25 minutes or until vegetables are tender, stirring occasionally.

*Makes 4 servings*

**TIP:** Choose parsnips that are firm, unblemished and small or medium in size (about 8 inches long). Rinse and scrub parsnips with a vegetable brush before using to remove embedded soil.

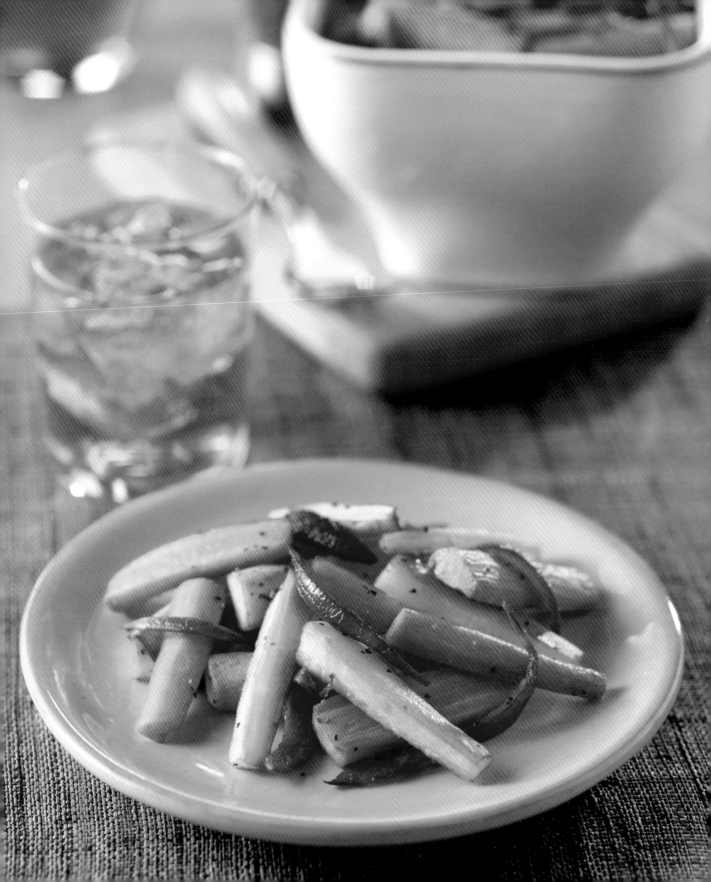

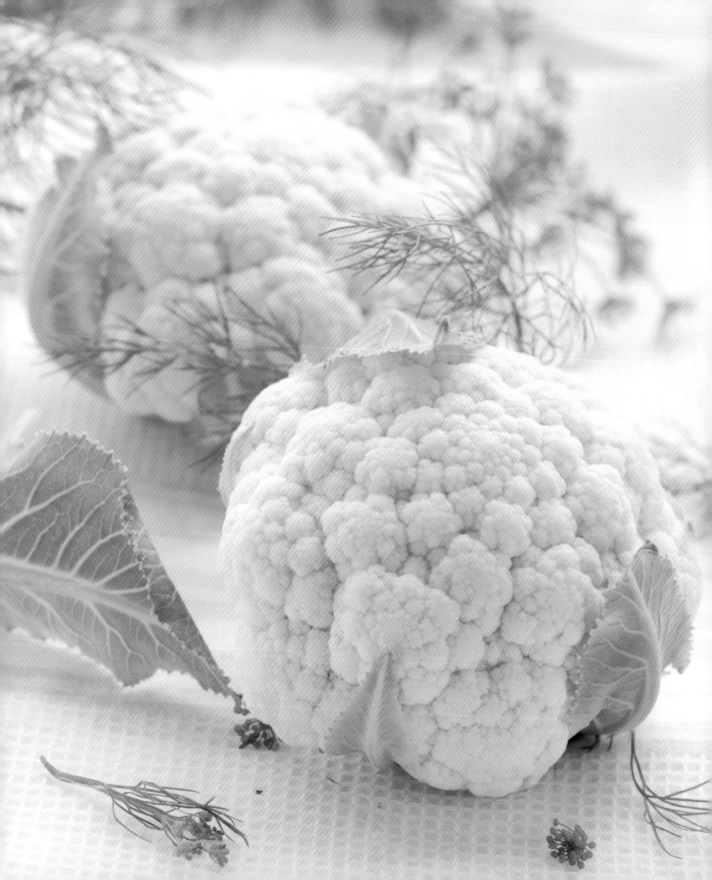

# CAULIFLOWER

High in fiber and low in calories, cauliflower is versatile enough to blend with and enhance flavors in a wide variety of dishes. This healthy cruciferous vegetable is a favorite in cuisines from Italy to India.

After citrus fruits, cauliflower is your next best natural source of vitamin C, an antioxidant vitamin with wide-ranging effects. Research suggests vitamin C may help defend blood vessels from damage and possibly slow the hardening of arteries that can lead to heart attack or stroke. It may also lower the risk of high blood pressure, arthritis, sight-stealing macular degeneration and asthma. Plus, the natural chemical that gives cauliflower its sharp taste may help protect against cancers of the breast and prostate. Cauliflower is also a good source of folate and potassium.

# CAULIFLOWER
# AND POTATO MASALA

2 tablespoons coconut oil

1 teaspoon minced garlic

1 teaspoon finely chopped
   fresh ginger

1 teaspoon salt

1 teaspoon cumin seeds

1 teaspoon ground coriander

1½ cups chopped tomatoes,
   fresh or canned

1 head cauliflower (about
   1¼ pounds), broken into
   florets

8 ounces medium red potatoes,
   peeled and cut into wedges

½ teaspoon garam masala

2 tablespoons chopped fresh
   cilantro

**1** Heat oil in large saucepan over medium-high heat. Add garlic, ginger, salt, cumin and coriander; cook and stir about 30 seconds or until fragrant.

**2** Add tomatoes; cook and stir 1 minute. Add cauliflower and potatoes; mix well. Reduce heat to low; cover and cook about 30 minutes or until vegetables are tender.

**3** Stir in garam masala; mix well. sprinkle with cilantro.

*Makes 6 servings*

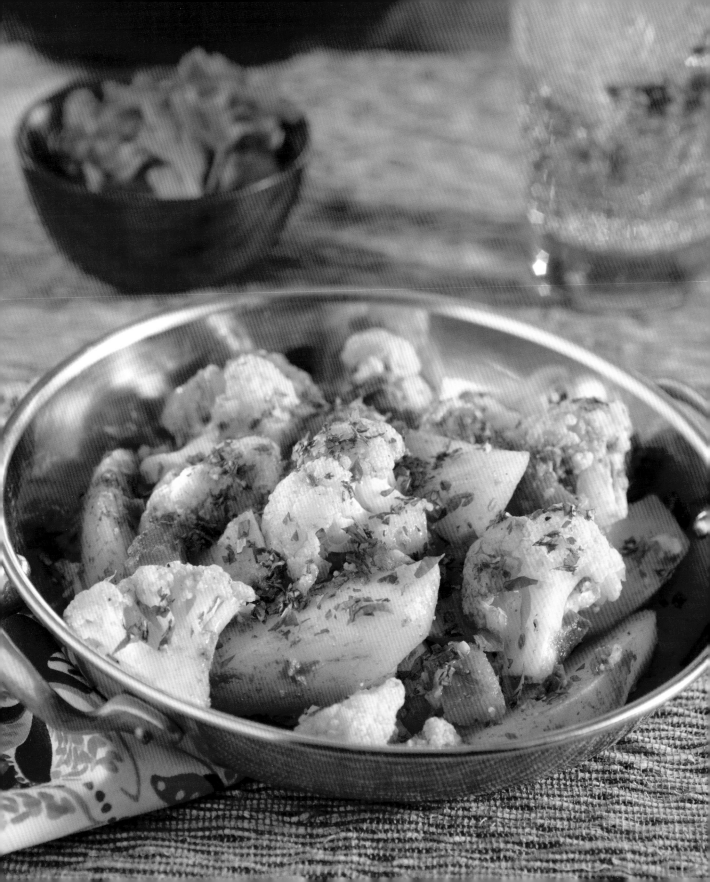

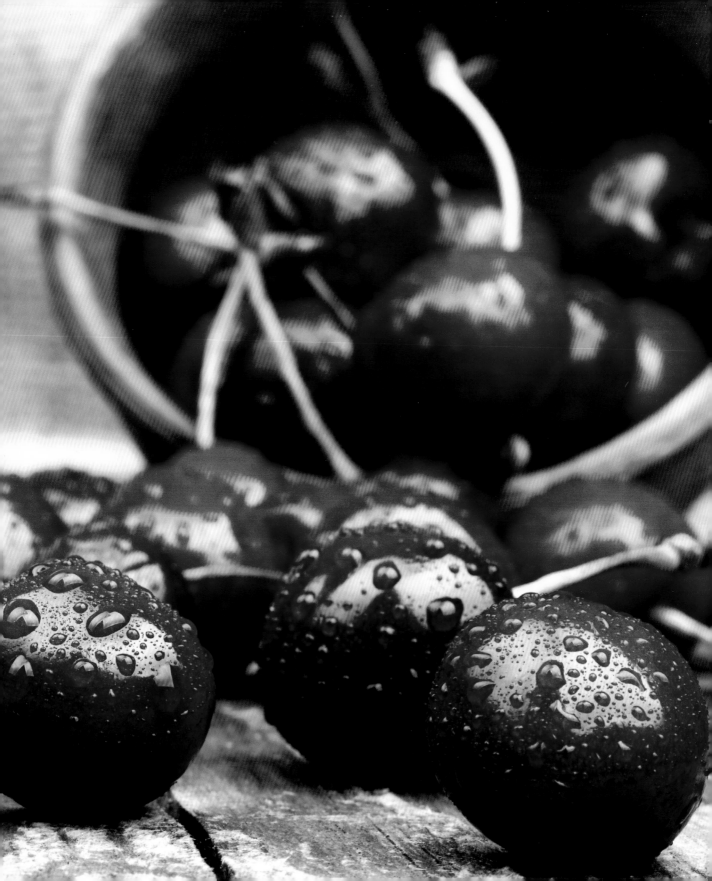

# CHERRIES

Cherry season might be short, but you can still enjoy cherries—and their powerful nutritional punch—all year long. Fresh, frozen, canned, dried or juiced, cherries may provide a range of important health benefits, from helping to ease the pain of arthritis and gout to reducing risk factors for heart disease, diabetes and certain cancers.

Compared to sweet cherries, tart (or sour) cherries are higher in vitamins and minerals, but both types provide disease-fighting antioxidants, including beta-carotene and vitamin C. Cherries supply potassium, which is essential for healthy blood pressure, and soluble fiber, which helps lower cholesterol and regulate blood sugar. Cherries also contain melatonin, which has been found to help regulate the body's natural sleep patterns and aid with jet lag. It may even play a role in preventing memory loss and delaying the aging process.

# FRUIT SALAD WITH CHERRY VINAIGRETTE

½ cup fresh cherries, pitted and chopped

¼ cup orange juice

2 tablespoons balsamic vinegar

1 to 2 tablespoons honey

1 tablespoon safflower oil

Pinch salt

3 cups diced cantaloupe

1 large mango, peeled and diced

¼ cup sliced almonds

**1** Combine cherries, orange juice, vinegar, honey, oil and salt in small bowl; mix well.

**2** Combine cantaloupe and mango in large bowl. Add dressing just before serving; toss to coat. Sprinkle with almonds.

*Makes 8 servings*

**TIP:** You can substitute peaches or nectarines for the mango. If fresh cherries are not available, use frozen cherries, thawed and well drained.

# CHERRY ALMOND SMOOTHIE

½ cup almond milk

1½ cups frozen dark sweet cherries

½ banana

2 teaspoons almond butter

⅛ teaspoon ground cinnamon

Combine almond milk, cherries, banana, almond butter and cinnamon in blender; blend until smooth.

*Makes 2 servings*

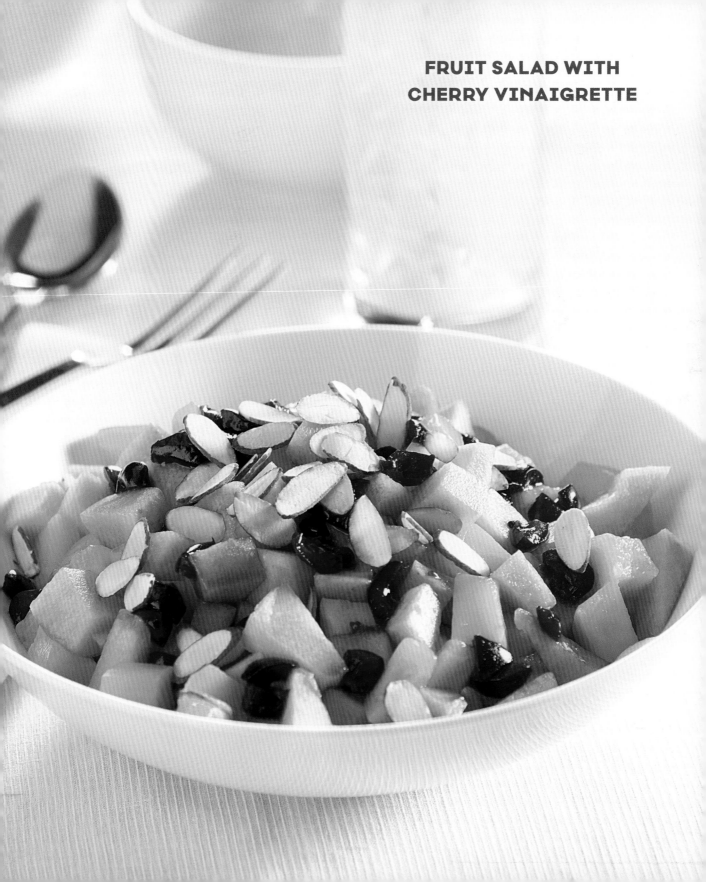

**FRUIT SALAD WITH
CHERRY VINAIGRETTE**

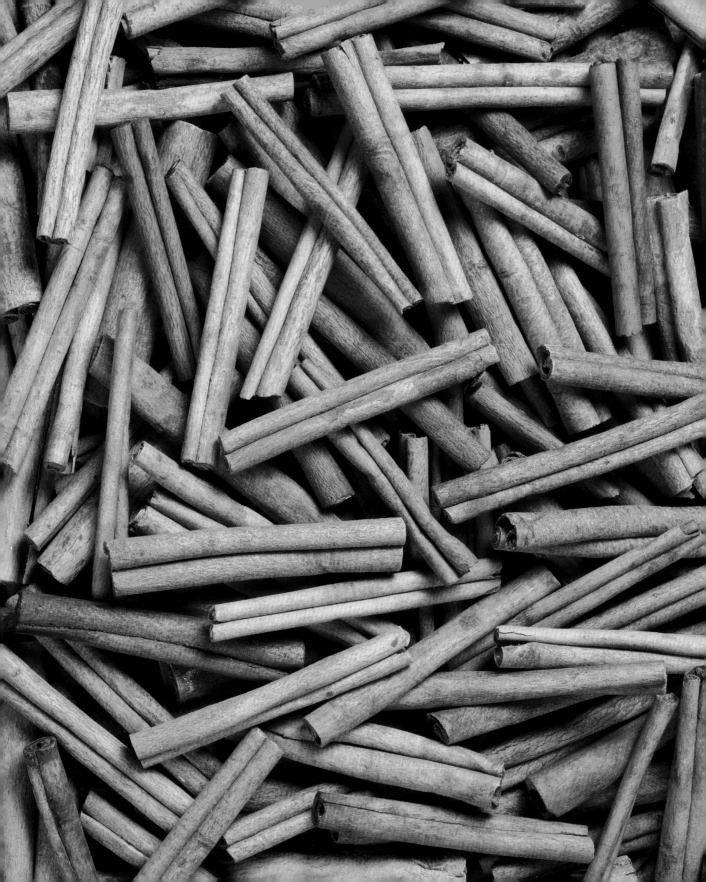

# CINNAMON

Used for centuries as for both cooking and medicinal purposes, cinnamon now shows promise in supporting overall health and wellness. Cinnamon has one of the highest antioxidant levels of any spice; it even has more than many foods. One teaspoon of cinnamon contains as many antioxidants as a full cup of pomegranate juice or ½ cup of blueberries.

Warming your diet with cinnamon feeds your immune system with antioxidant fuel for the fight against infection and disease. And according to several studies, a mere ½ teaspoon of cinnamon daily can improve insulin sensitivity, which in turn can help lower diabetes and heart disease risk. Cinnamon may also help lower blood cholesterol and triglyceride levels, relieve bloating and gas, and reduce heartburn discomfort.

# MIDDLE EASTERN VEGETABLE STEW

¼ **cup olive oil**

3 **cups (12 ounces) sliced zucchini**

2 **cups (6 ounces) cubed peeled eggplant**

2 **cups sliced quartered peeled sweet potatoes**

1½ **cups cubed peeled butternut squash**

1 **can (28 ounces) crushed tomatoes in purée**

1 **cup drained canned chickpeas**

½ **cup raisins or currants (optional)**

1½ **teaspoons ground cinnamon**

1 **teaspoon grated orange peel**

¾ **teaspoon ground cumin**

½ **teaspoon salt**

½ **teaspoon paprika**

¼ **to ½ teaspoon ground red pepper**

⅛ **teaspoon ground cardamom**

**Hot cooked whole wheat couscous or brown rice (optional)**

**1** Heat oil in large saucepan or Dutch oven over medium heat. Add zucchini, eggplant, sweet potatoes and squash; cook and stir 8 to 10 minutes or until vegetables are slightly softened.

**2** Stir in tomatoes, chickpeas, raisins, if desired, cinnamon, orange peel, cumin, salt, paprika, red pepper and cardamom; bring to a boil over high heat. Reduce heat to low; cover and cook 30 minutes or until vegetables are tender. If sauce becomes too thick, stir in water to thin.

**3** Serve over couscous, if desired.

*Makes 6 servings*

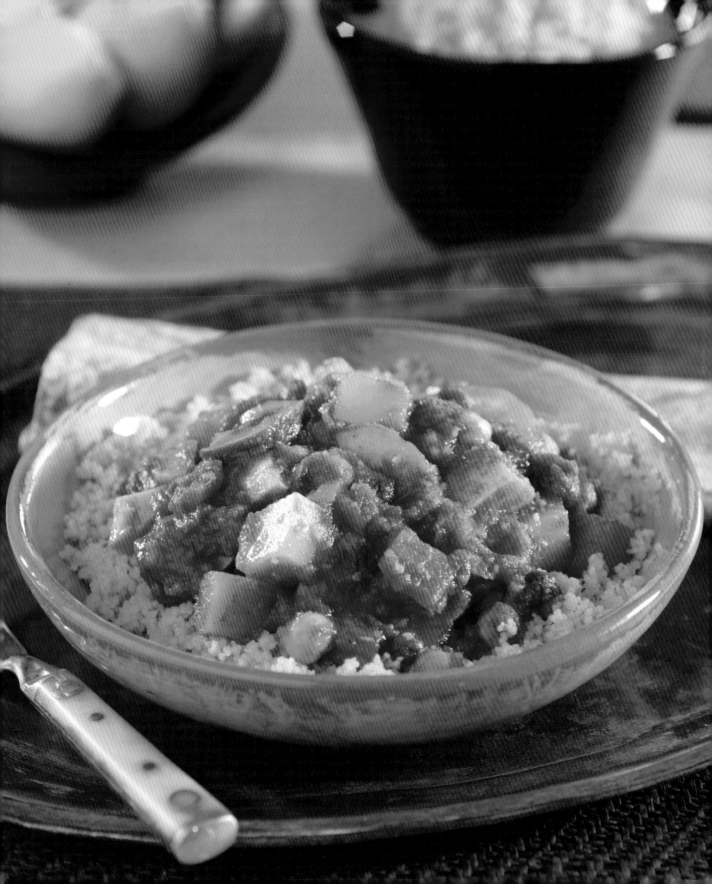

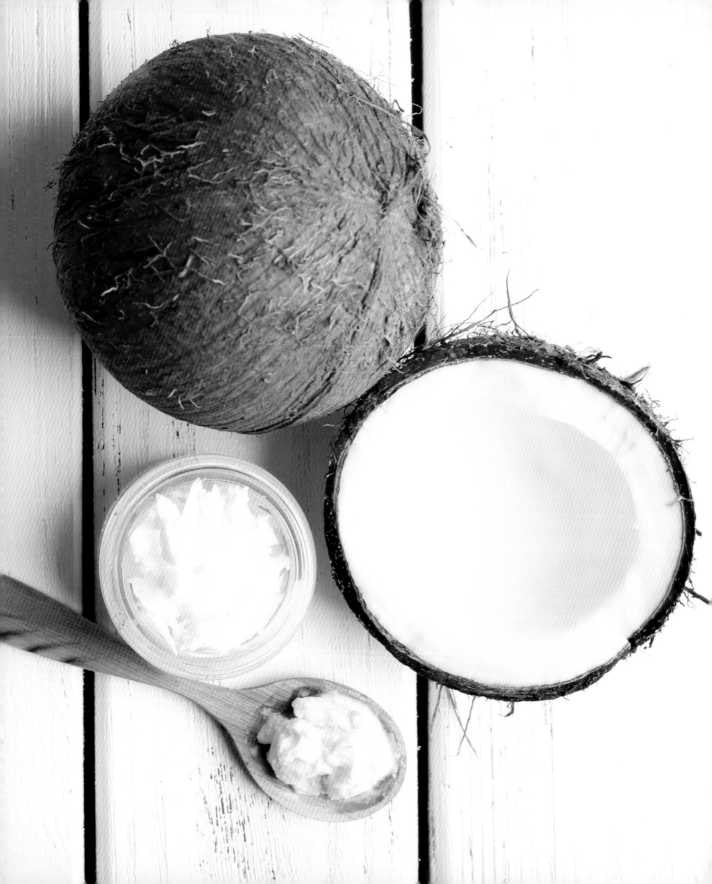

# COCONUT

Classified as a seed, a fruit and a nut, the versatile coconut produces a wide array of products including coconut water, coconut cream, coconut milk, coconut oil, and of course, coconut meat.

Coconuts contain beneficial dietary fats that may help protect the heart and prevent cardiovascular disease. They are thought to increase the levels of HDL's ("good" cholesterol) and lower the level of LDL's ("bad" cholesterol), and they may also help lower blood pressure. Coconut oil has been shown to contain saturated fatty acids with antibacterial and antiviral properties, while coconut meat and milk are high in dietary fiber, minerals and protein.

# THAI VEGGIE CURRY

4 tablespoons coconut oil, divided

2 sweet potatoes, peeled and cut into thin strips or spiralized

1 onion, cut into thin strips or spiralized

1 tablespoon Thai red curry paste (or to taste)

1 can (about 13 ounces) unsweetened light coconut milk

2 red or yellow bell peppers, cut into thin strips or spiralized

1½ cups cauliflower and/or broccoli florets

1 cup snow peas

1 package (about 14 ounces) tofu, pressed* and cubed

Salt and black pepper

¼ cup slivered fresh basil

*Cut tofu in half horizontally and place it between layers of paper towels. Place a weighted cutting board on top; let stand 15 to 30 minutes.

1 Heat 2 tablespoons oil in large skillet over medium heat. Add sweet potatoes; cook and stir 10 to 15 minutes or until sweet potatoes are tender. Transfer to medium bowl; cover to keep warm.

2 Heat remaining 2 tablespoons oil in same skillet over medium heat. Add onion; cook and stir 3 minutes or until softened. Add curry paste; cook and stir 1 minute. Add coconut milk; bring to a boil, stirring to dissove curry paste.

3 Add bell peppers and cauliflower; cook 4 to 5 minutes or until crisp-tender. Stir in snow peas; cook 2 minutes.

4 Gently stir in tofu; cook until heated through. Season with salt and black pepper. Sprinkle with basil; serve curry over sweet potatoes.

*Makes 4 to 6 servings*

**VARIATION:** Substitute any other vegetables for the cauliflower and snow peas. Try frozen peas, baby corn, carrots or zucchini.

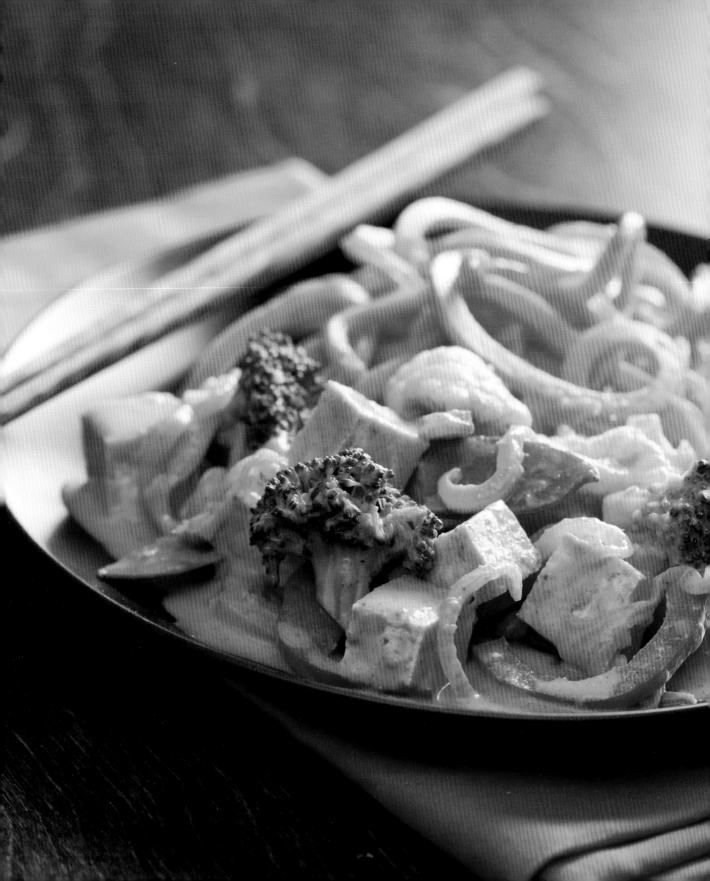

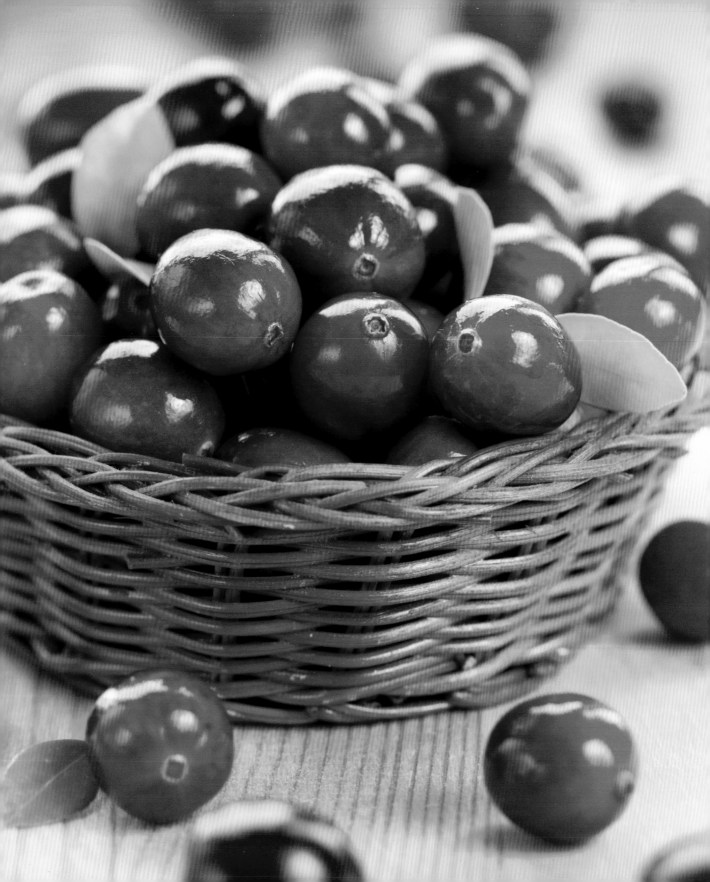

# CRANBERRIES

Tart and tangy cranberries are another popular seasonal fruit that deserves to be enjoyed year round. They bring brilliant color and flavor to both sweet and savory dishes, and they provide great health benefits in any form (fresh, frozen, dried or juiced).

Cranberries contain phytonutrients that prevent certain bacteria from sticking to the walls of the urinary tract, thus helping to prevent or treat urinary tract infections and interstitial cystitis (a condition resulting in bladder and pelvic discomfort). This same antibacterial effect may also help prevent gum disease and stomach ulcers, both commonly caused by bacteria. In addition, cranberries contain fiber as well as significant amounts of antioxidants and other phytonutrients that may help protect against heart disease, cancer and eye diseases.

# BROWN RICE WITH CRANBERRIES AND WALNUTS

1 **can (about 14 ounces) vegetable or chicken broth**

¾ **cup uncooked brown rice or brown basmati rice**

¼ **cup water**

¼ **teaspoon salt**

¼ **cup dried cranberries**

⅛ **teaspoon ground cinnamon**

¼ **cup coarsely chopped walnuts, toasted***

*\*To toast walnuts, spread on baking sheet. Bake in preheated 350°F oven 6 to 8 minutes or until golden brown, stirring frequently.*

1 Combine broth, rice, water and salt in large saucepan; bring to a boil over high heat. Reduce heat to low; cover and simmer 20 minutes.

2 Stir in cranberries and cinnamon; cover and simmer 20 to 25 minutes or until rice is tender. Sprinkle with walnuts just before serving.

*Makes 4 servings*

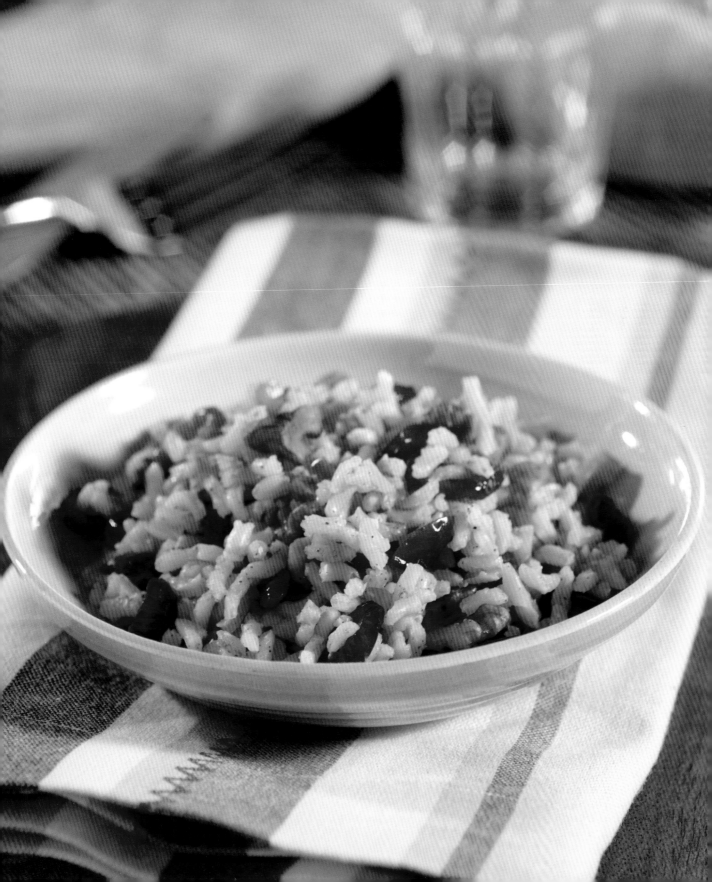

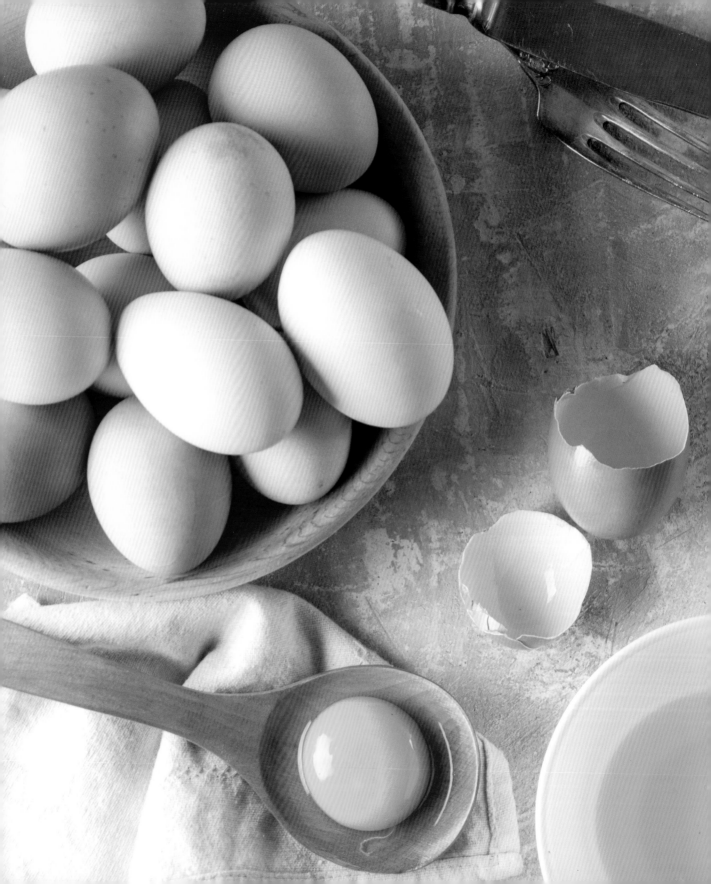

# EGGS

Eggs are one of nature's most perfect nutrient packages, complete with 13 essential vitamins and minerals, high-quality protein, healthy unsaturated fats and protective antioxidants—all for about 75 calories. Incredible!

Although eggs are high in cholesterol, they are fairly low in fat, and evidence consistently shows that eating one or more eggs each day does not increase heart disease risk in healthy adults and may actually be associated with lower blood pressure. Eggs are a good source of the antioxidants lutein and zeaxanthin that, according to many studies, reduce the risk of sight-stealing cataracts and macular degeneration in older adults. Eggs also provide a third to half of the daily need for choline, a vitamin essential for brain development in fetuses and infants that may also help prevent age-related memory loss and promote liver and heart health.

# EDAMAME FRITTATA

2   tablespoons olive oil

½   cup frozen shelled edamame

⅓   cup frozen corn

¼   cup chopped shallot (1 shallot)

5   eggs

¾   teaspoon Italian seasoning

½   teaspoon salt

½   teaspoon black pepper

¼   cup chopped green onions

½   cup crumbled goat cheese

**1** Preheat broiler. Heat oil in large broilerproof skillet over medium-high heat. Add edamame, corn and shallot; cook and stir 6 to 8 minutes or until shallot is browned and edamame are hot.

**2** Meanwhile, beat eggs, Italian seasoning, salt and pepper in medium bowl until blended. Stir in green onions. Pour egg mixture over vegetables in skillet; sprinkle with cheese. Cook over medium heat 5 to 7 minutes or until eggs are set on bottom, lifting up mixture to allow uncooked portion to flow underneath.

**3** Broil 6 inches from heat 1 minute or until top is puffy and golden. Loosen frittata from skillet with spatula; slide onto small platter. Cut into wedges.

***Makes 4 servings***

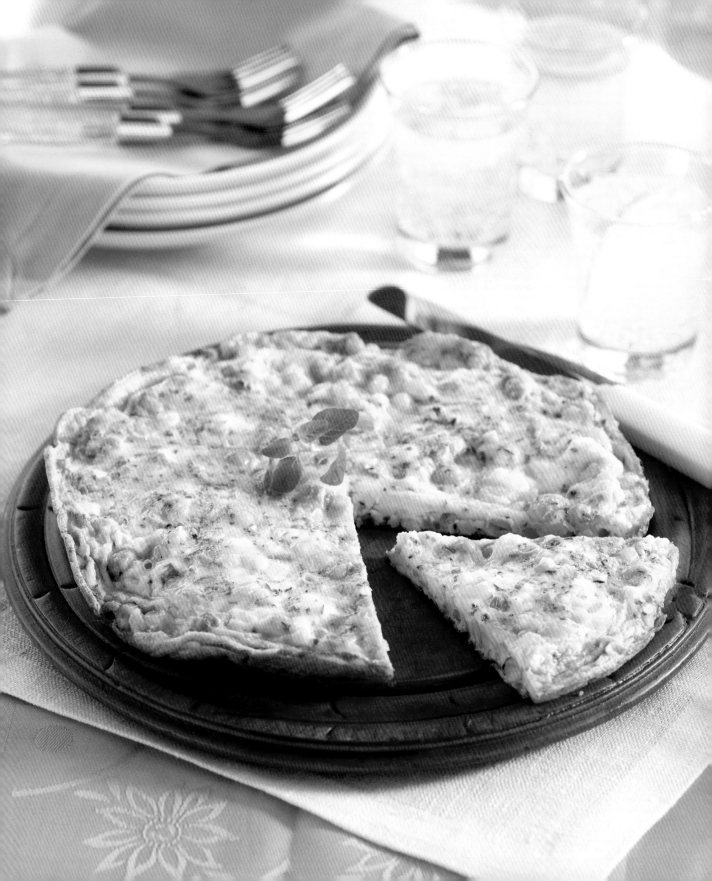

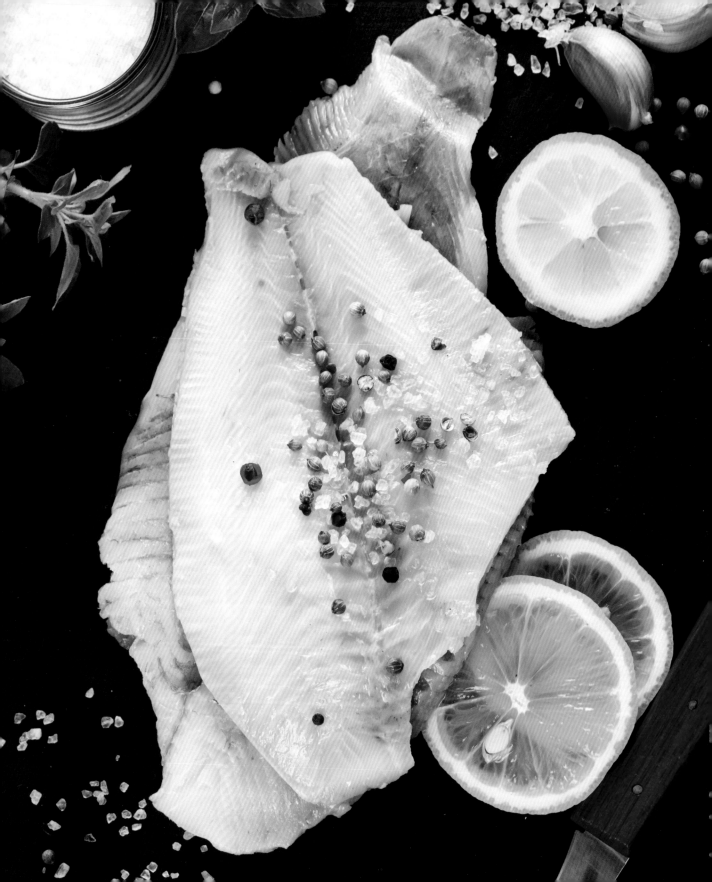

# FISH

High in protein and low in saturated fat, fish is a smart catch for a healthy diet. Health experts recommend eating fish at least twice a week—it provides quality protein on par with meat but generally contains less total and saturated fat than even the leanest cuts of beef or chicken.

Fish contains omega-3 fatty acids, good unsaturated fats that help prevent heart disease and cancer, treat arthritis, reduce inflammation and depression and improve memory. Fatty fishes, such as salmon, mackerel, sardines, anchovies, trout, tuna, whitefish, bass, ocean perch and halibut, are higher in omega-3s.

# GRILLED RED SNAPPER WITH AVOCADO-PAPAYA SALSA

1 teaspoon ground coriander

1 teaspoon paprika

¾ teaspoon salt

⅛ to ¼ teaspoon ground
   red pepper

½ cup diced ripe avocado

½ cup diced ripe papaya

2 tablespoons chopped
   fresh cilantro

1 tablespoon lime juice

1 tablespoon olive oil

4 skinless red snapper or halibut
   fillets (5 to 7 ounces each)

4 lime wedges

**1** Prepare grill for direct cooking. Oil grid. Combine coriander, paprika, salt and red pepper in small bowl; mix well.

**2** For salsa, combine avocado, papaya, cilantro, lime juice and ¼ teaspoon coriander mixture in medium bowl; mix well.

**3** Brush oil over fish; sprinkle with remaining coriander mixture.

**4** Grill fish, covered, over medium-high heat 10 minutes or until fish begins to flake when tested with fork, turning once. Serve with salsa and lime wedges.

*Makes 4 servings*

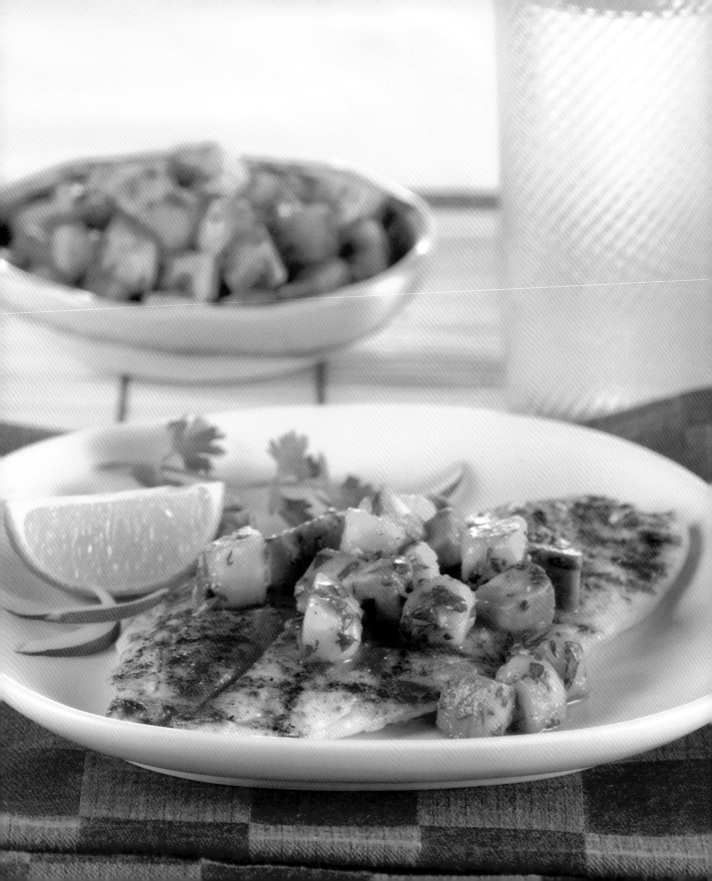

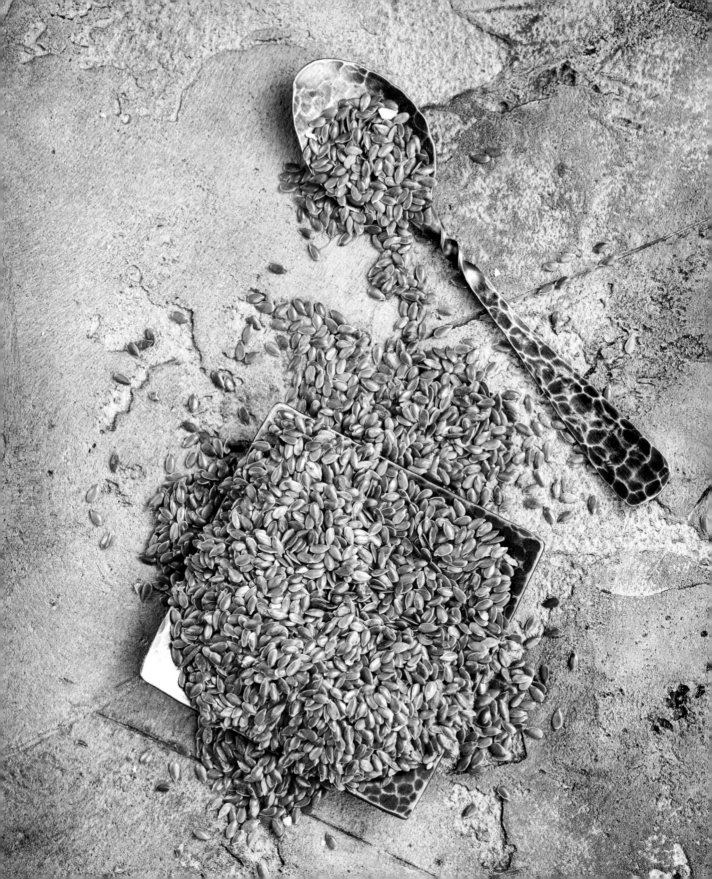

# FLAXSEED

A small seed with enormous health benefits, flax seed can be used in everything from meat loaves and muffins to smoothies and cereal. Flaxseed may be purchased whole or ground, but to unlock its potential benefits, flaxseed must be ground before eating.

Flaxseed is packed with soluble fiber, the kind that helps lower blood cholesterol levels and helps keep blood sugar levels steady. Flaxseed is also rich in antioxidants and phytonutrients that may play a role in warding off breast cancer and protecting the intestines in those with inflammatory bowel disease. Flaxseed is best known for providing a healthy dose of alpha linolenic acid, the plant version of omega-3 fatty acids (an essential polyunsaturated fat the body cannot make for itself). This form of unsaturated fat helps to fight inflammation that can lead to heart disease, cancer, diabetes and arthritis.

# QUINOA AND OAT MUESLI

1 cup uncooked quinoa

3 cups old-fashioned oats

¼ cup unsweetened flaked
 coconut

¾ cup coarsely chopped almonds

½ teaspoon ground cinnamon

½ cup toasted wheat germ

¼ cup ground flaxseeds

1¼ cups chopped dried fruit

1 Preheat oven to 350°F. Spread quinoa on baking sheet. Bake 8 to 10 minutes until toasted and golden brown, stirring frequently. (Quinoa will make a slight popping sound when almost done.) Transfer to small bowl; cool completely.

2 Combine oats, coconut, almonds and cinnamon in large bowl; mix well. Spread in even layer on same baking sheet. Bake 15 minutes or until mixture is toasted and fragrant. Cool completely.

3 Combine cooled quinoa and oat mixture in large bowl; stir in wheat germ, flaxseeds and dried fruit until blended.

***Makes 6¾ cups***

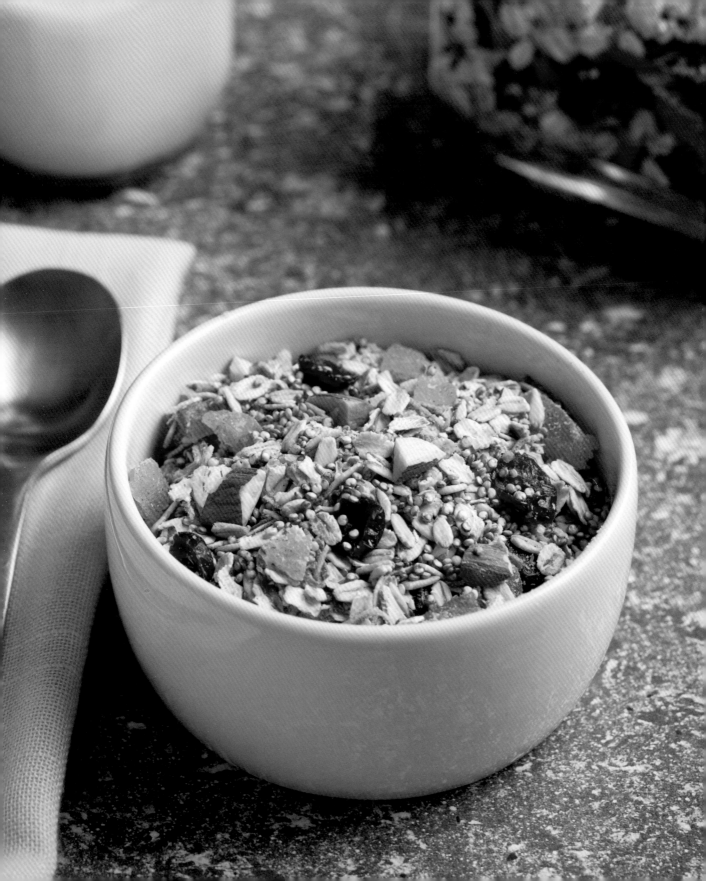

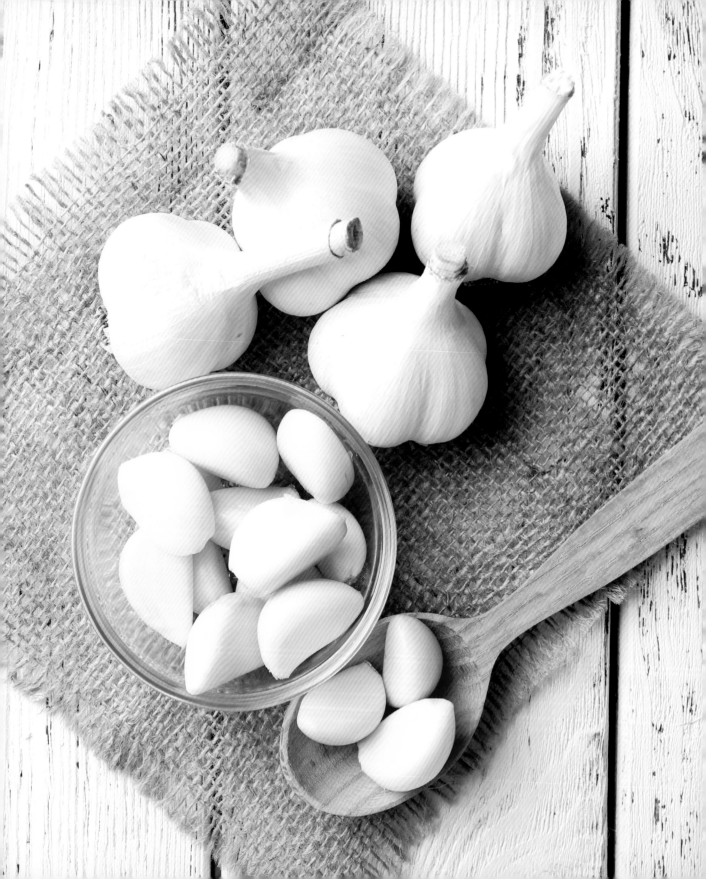

# GARLIC

Garlic has been grown for more than 5,000 years, and ancient cultures believed that it had incredible powers—to keep away evil spirits, to enhance strength, to treat wounds and to ease digestive disorders. Modern science has confirmed that raw garlic has antibacterial and antiviral properties.

When garlic is crushed, finely chopped or cooked, a substance called allicin is formed, providing garlic's distinctive aroma and flavor. Research suggests this compound can help lower high blood pressure and slow the hardening of arteries that can lead to heart attacks and strokes. Eating garlic also seems to lower the risk of stomach, colon and rectal cancers. And it may be effective at killing bacteria and reducing colds.

# FORTY-CLOVE CHICKEN FILICE

¼ **cup olive oil**

1 **whole chicken (about 3 pounds), cut into serving pieces**

40 **cloves garlic (about 2 heads), peeled**

4 **stalks celery, thickly sliced**

½ **cup dry white wine**

¼ **cup dry vermouth**

**Grated peel and juice of 1 lemon**

2 **tablespoons finely chopped fresh parsley**

2 **teaspoons dried basil**

1 **teaspoon dried oregano**

**Pinch of red pepper flakes**

**Salt and black pepper**

**1** Preheat oven to 375°F.

**2** Heat oil in Dutch oven over medium-high heat. Add chicken; cook until browned on all sides.

**3** Combine garlic, celery, wine, vermouth, lemon juice, parsley, basil, oregano and red pepper flakes in medium bowl; pour over chicken. Sprinkle with lemon peel; season with salt and black pepper.

**4** Cover and bake 40 minutes. Uncover; bake 15 minutes or until chicken is cooked through (165°F).

***Makes 4 to 6 servings***

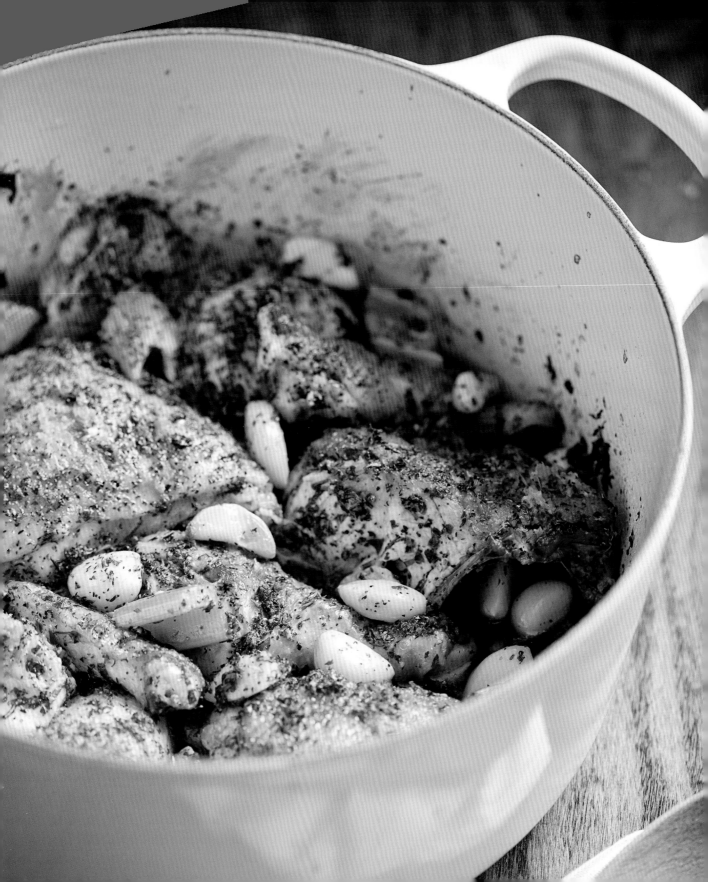

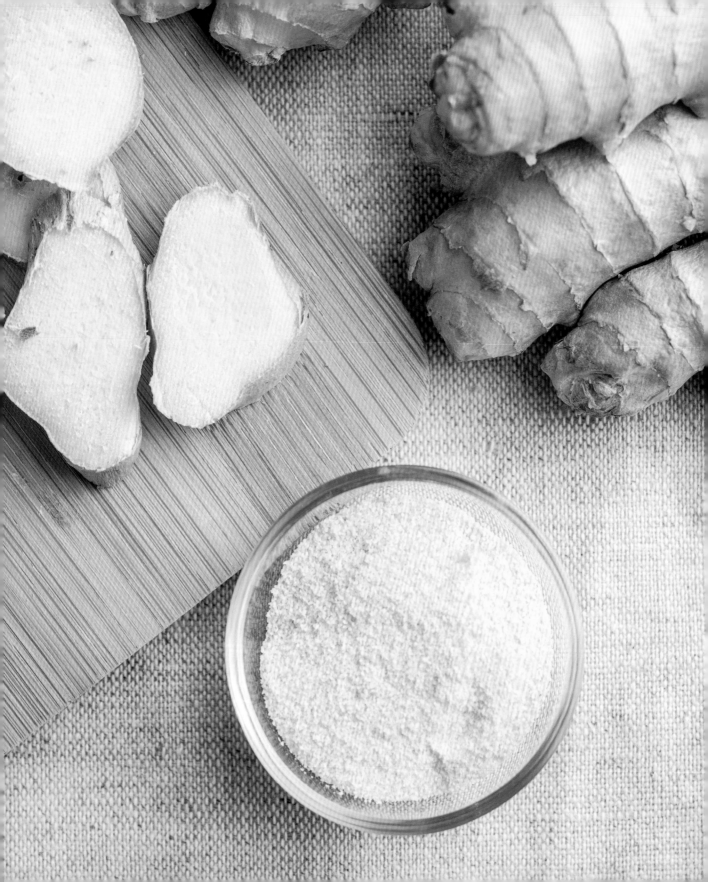

# GINGER

Aromatic and spicy, ginger has been valued for its culinary and medicinal properties for thousands of years. Ginger has traditionally been used as a remedy for gastrointestinal upset, and research supports its use for alleviating the symptoms of motion sickness, morning sickness related to pregnancy and even nausea associated with chemotherapy.

Ginger is also rich in antioxidant substances that have anti-inflammatory effects, which may explain its apparent ability to reduce joint pain, swelling and stiffness in people with arthritis. Ginger's anti-inflammatory effects may also prove beneficial in combating cancer, heart disease and the growing list of other diseases linked to chronic inflammation in the body. Substances in ginger called gingerols have antimicrobial and antifungal properties that help fight infections and boost your immunity.

# CHILI GINGER SHRIMP

1 tablespoon plus 2 teaspoons soy sauce, divided

1½ tablespoons safflower oil, divided

2 teaspoons grated fresh ginger

2 teaspoons lemon juice, divided

1 pound raw jumbo shrimp, peeled and deveined

2 tablespoons chili garlic sauce

⅛ teaspoon black pepper

Hot cooked rice (optional)

2 tablespoons minced fresh cilantro

**1** Combine 1 tablespoon soy sauce, ½ tablespoon oil, ginger and 1 teaspoon lemon juice in large bowl. Add shrimp; toss to coat. Cover and refrigerate 1 hour.

**2** Combine chili garlic sauce, remaining 2 teaspoons soy sauce, 1 teaspoon lemon juice and pepper in small bowl; mix well.

**3** Heat remaining 1 tablespoon oil in large skillet over medium-high heat. Drain shrimp, reserving marinade. Add shrimp to skillet; stir-fry 6 minutes or until shrimp are pink and opaque.

**4** Add reserved marinade and chili garlic sauce mixture to skillet; cook and stir 1 minute or until sauce boils and thickens slightly. Serve over rice, if desired. Sprinkle with cilantro.

*Makes 4 servings*

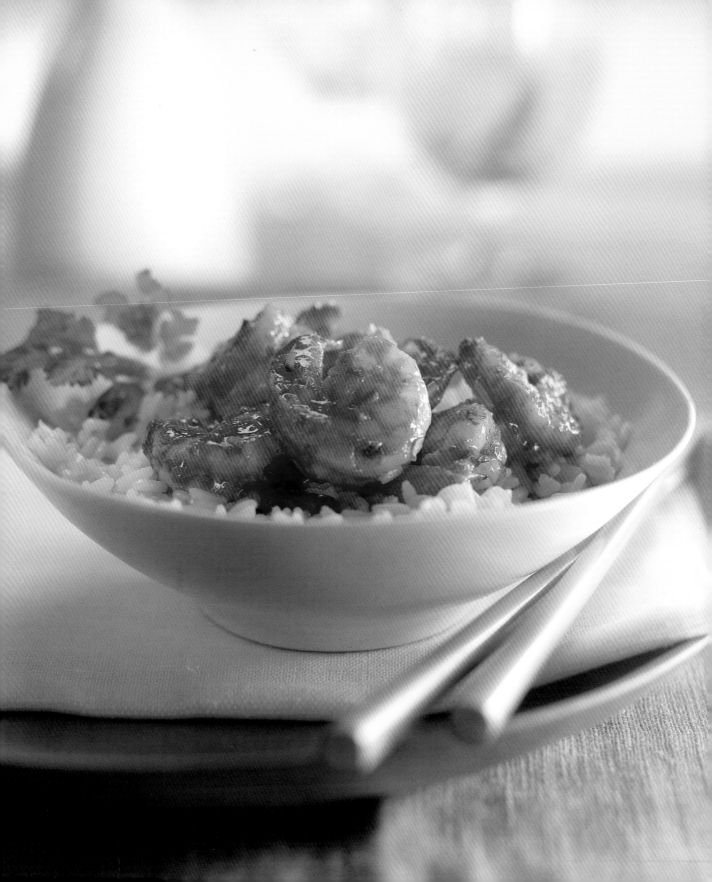

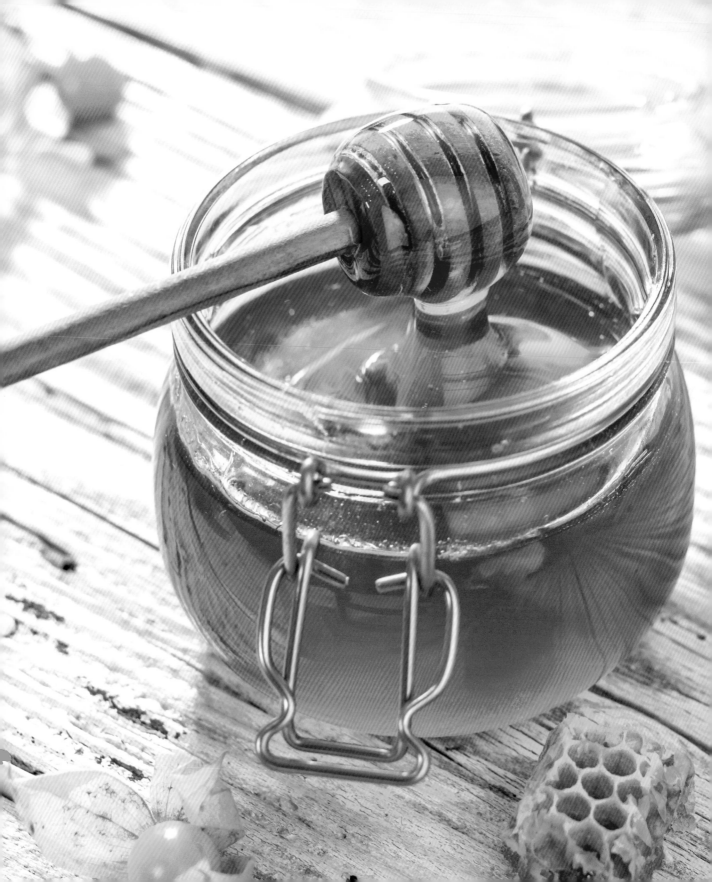

# HONEY

This natural sweetener is a treasure trove of nutritional and medicinal benefits, used since the days of the ancient Egyptians.

Honey helps suppress coughs and sooth sore throats, while honey's anti-inflammatory properties make it a good natural option to reduce the irritation and itch from insect bites. Honey is packed with polyphenols, a type of antioxidant that can help protect cells from damage caused by free radicals. Honey's ability to help the body absorb calcium helps to aid brain health. And honey may help improve cholesterol levels, reducing total and LDL cholesterol while raising HDL cholesterol levels. It may also help lower triglyceride levels, which can reduce the risk for heart disease and type 2 diabetes.

# SKILLET ROASTED ROOT VEGETABLES

1   **sweet potato, peeled, cut in half lengthwise and then cut crosswise into ½-inch slices**

1   **large red onion, cut into 1-inch wedges**

2   **parsnips, cut diagonally into 1-inch slices**

2   **carrots, cut diagonally into 1-inch slices**

1   **turnip, peeled, cut in half and then cut into ½-inch slices**

2½   **tablespoons olive oil**

1½   **tablespoons honey**

1½   **tablespoons balsamic vinegar**

1   **teaspoon coarse salt**

1   **teaspoon dried thyme**

¼   **teaspoon ground red pepper**

¼   **teaspoon black pepper**

**1**  Preheat oven to 400°F.

**2**  Combine all ingredients in large bowl; toss to coat. Spread vegetables in single layer in large cast iron skillet.

**3**  Roast 1 hour or until vegetables are tender, stirring once halfway through cooking time.

*Makes 4 servings*

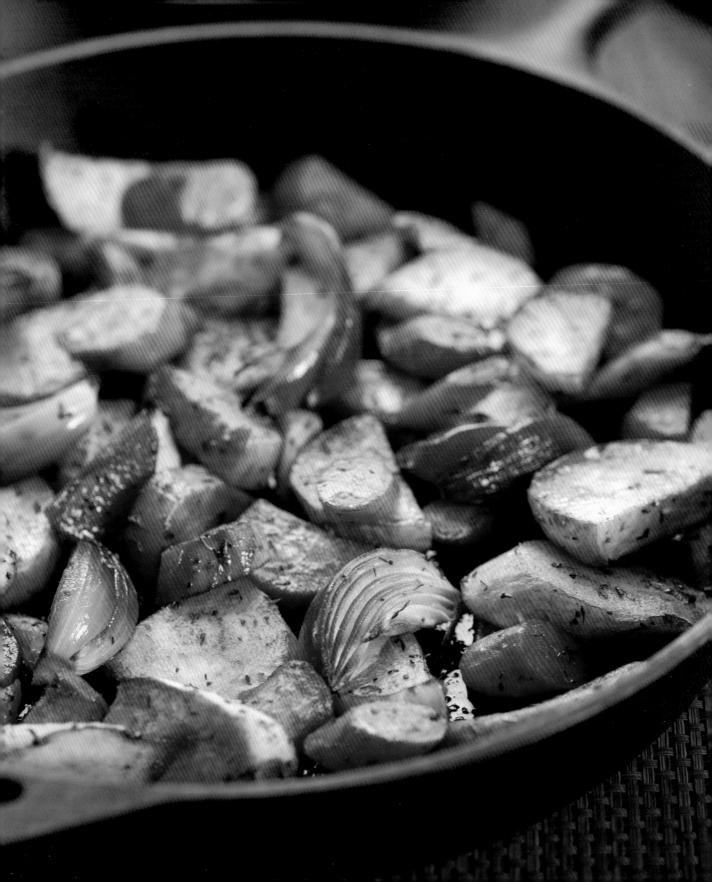

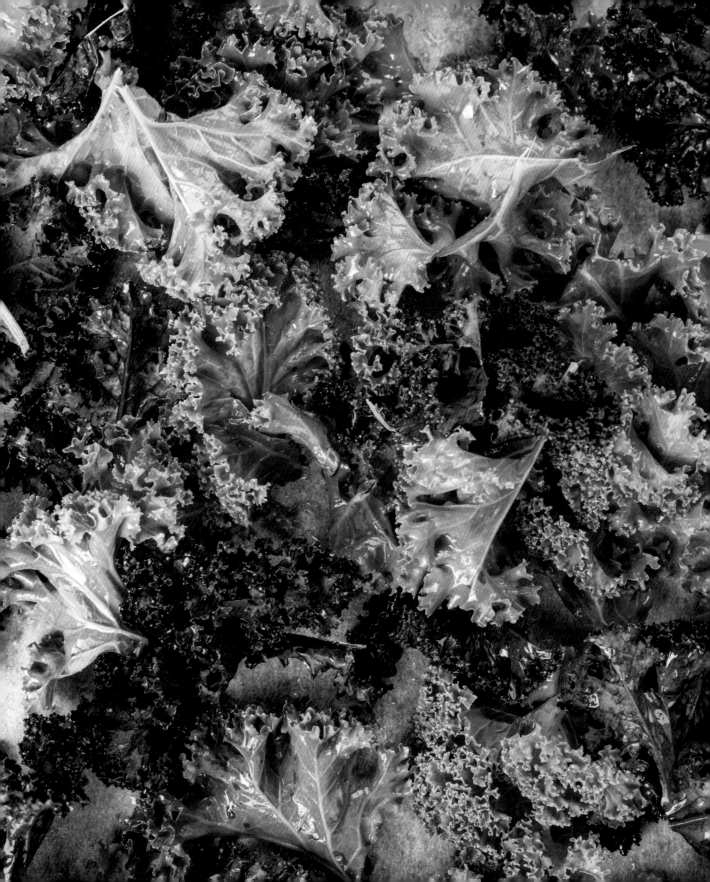

# KALE

Kale might be the most popular member of the cabbage family—a true nutrient-dense superfood.

Kale stands a head above other greens as an excellent source of beta-carotene and vitamin C, two antioxidants believed to be major players in the body's battle against cancer, heart disease and certain age-related chronic diseases. Kale is also a phenomenal source of readily absorbed calcium, a mineral that is vital to warding off osteoporosis, may reduce symptoms of premenstrual syndrome and may help keep blood pressure in a healthy range. Kale contains an enormous amount of vitamin K, which promotes brain and bone health, while the fiber and sulfur in kale aid with digestion and liver health. Kale also provides iron, folate, vitamin B6 and potassium.

# BULGUR PILAF WITH CARAMELIZED ONIONS AND KALE

1 tablespoon olive oil

1 small onion, cut into thin wedges

1 clove garlic, minced

2 cups chopped kale

2 cups vegetable or chicken broth

¾ cup medium grain bulgur

½ teaspoon salt

¼ teaspoon black pepper

**1** Heat oil in large nonstick skillet over medium heat. Add onion; cook about 8 minutes or until softened and lightly browned, stirring occasionally. Add garlic; cook and stir 1 minute.

**2** Add kale; cook and stir 1 to 2 minutes or until kale is wilted.

**3** Stir in broth, bulgur, salt and pepper; bring to a boil. Reduce heat to low; cover and cook 12 minutes or until liquid is absorbed and bulgur is tender.

*Makes 6 servings*

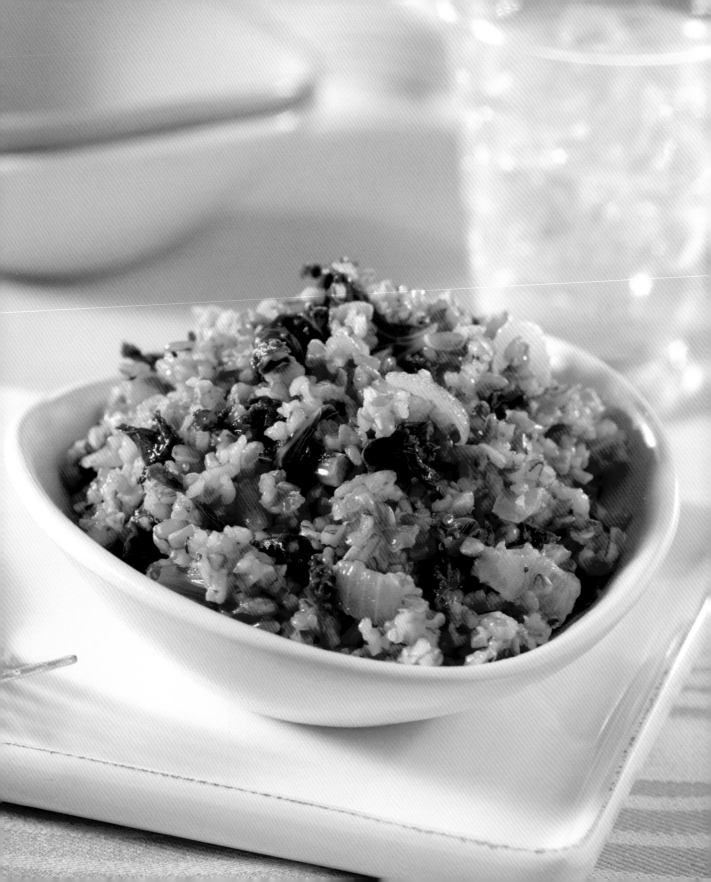

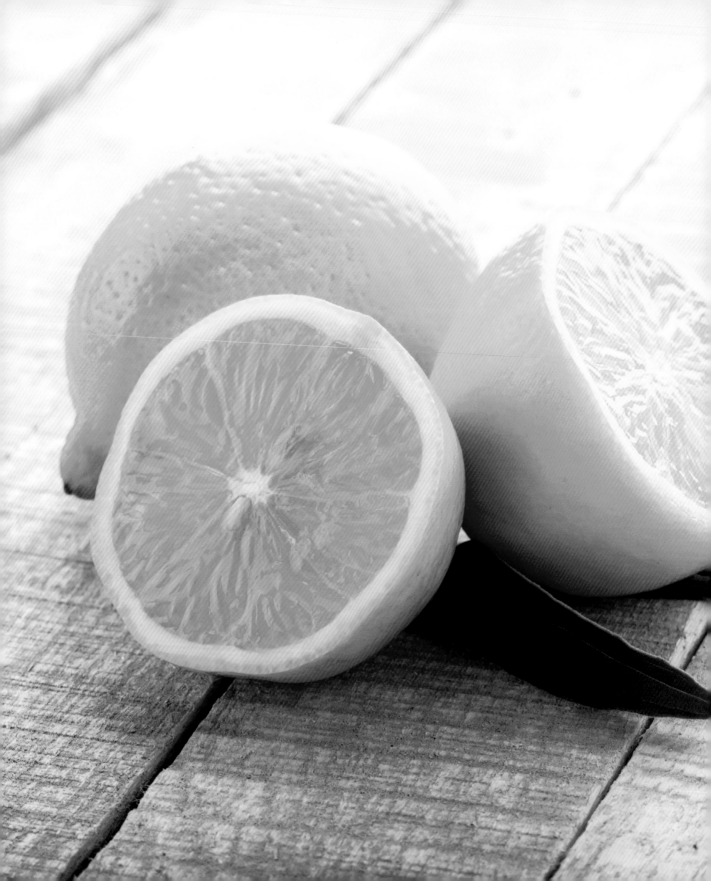

# LEMONS

Lemons add bright flavor to just about everything, appreciated in cuisines around the world for adding zest to both the savory and the sweet.

Lemons are loaded with vitamin C, a nutrient the body needs to heal wounds, control infections and make collagen, a protein the body uses to grow and repair blood vessels, skin, cartilage, ligaments, tendons, bones and teeth. Vitamin C is also an antioxidant that helps fight off heart disease, inflammation and cancer. The lemon's outer peel, or zest, is rich in yet another antioxidant called rutin, which may further help protect against heart disease by helping to strengthen blood vessel walls and protect them from damage.

# LEMON ROSEMARY SHRIMP AND VEGETABLE SOUVLAKI

8 ounces large raw shrimp, peeled and deveined (with tails on)

1 medium zucchini, halved lengthwise and cut into ½-inch slices

½ medium red bell pepper, cut into 1-inch pieces

8 green onions, trimmed and cut into 2-inch pieces

3 tablespoons extra virgin olive oil, divided

2 tablespoons lemon juice

2 teaspoons grated lemon peel

2 cloves garlic, minced

½ teaspoon salt

½ teaspoon chopped fresh rosemary

⅛ teaspoon red pepper flakes

1 Prepare grill for direct cooking. Oil grid or spray grill pan with nonstick cooking spray.

2 Spray four 12-inch bamboo or metal skewers with cooking spray. Alternately thread shrimp, zucchini, bell pepper and green onions onto skewers. Brush skewers lightly with 1 tablespoon oil.

3 Combine remaining 2 tablespoons oil, lemon juice, lemon peel, garlic, salt, rosemary and red pepper flakes in small bowl; mix well.

4 Grill skewers over high heat 2 minutes per side. Remove to serving platter; drizzle with sauce.

*Makes 4 servings*

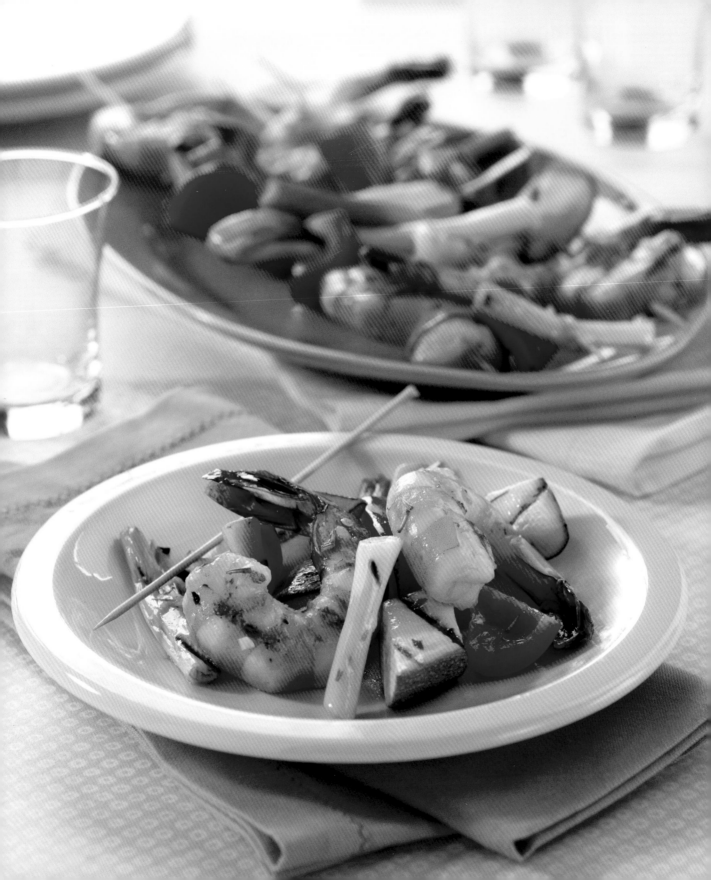

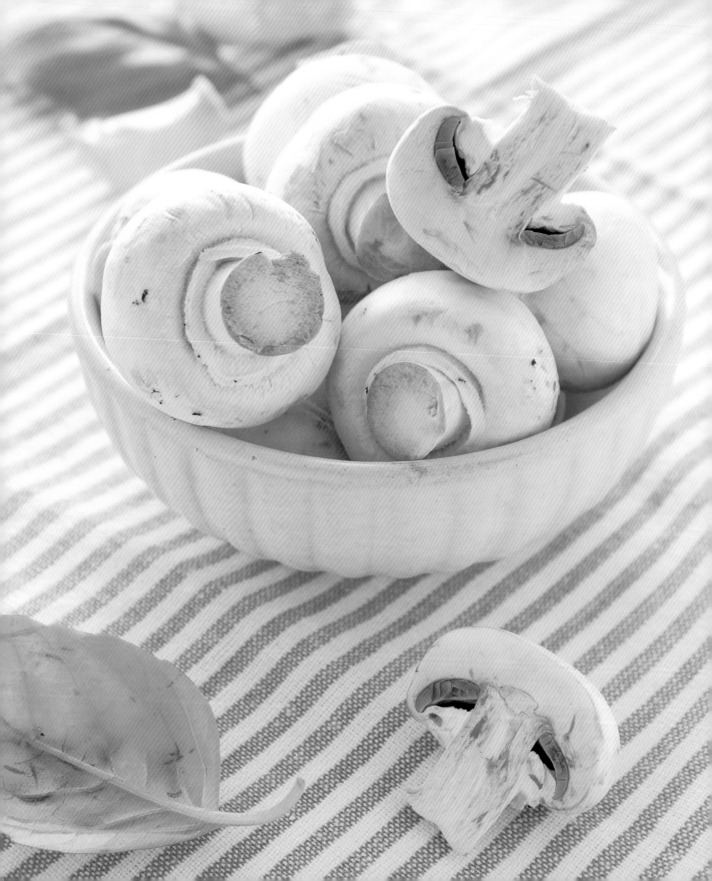

# MUSHROOMS

Despite their meaty texture and rich, earthy flavor, mushrooms are surprisingly low in calories, carbohydrates, fat and sodium.

Mushrooms provide important nutrients, including B vitamins and a large amount of potassium, which helps lower blood pressure. Mushrooms are the only plant source of vitamin D, naturally producing the vitamin following exposure to sunlight. Vitamin D is essential for bone health and is also being studied for its role in weight loss, as well as the prevention of cancer, heart disease and diabetes. Many varieties of mushrooms are also rich in selenium, an antioxidant mineral with anticancer properties.

# WILD MUSHROOM QUINOA STUFFING

1 cup uncooked quinoa

2 tablespoons olive oil, divided

2 cups vegetable broth

1 teaspoon poultry seasoning

½ teaspoon salt

1 small onion, diced

8 ounces cremini mushrooms, sliced

8 ounces shiitake mushrooms, stemmed and sliced

½ cup diced celery

2 tablespoons chopped fresh parsley (optional)

**1** Place quinoa in fine-mesh strainer; rinse well under cold running water.

**2** Heat 1 tablespoon oil in medium saucepan over medium-high heat. Add quinoa; stir until coated. Stir in broth, poultry seasoning and salt; bring to a boil. Reduce heat to low; cover and simmer 15 to 20 minutes or until quinoa is tender and broth is absorbed. Remove from heat.

**3** Meanwhile, heat remaining 1 tablespoon oil in large skillet over medium heat. Add onion, mushrooms and celery; cook and stir 8 to 10 minutes or until mushrooms begin to brown.

**4** Combine quinoa and vegetables in large bowl. Sprinkle with parsley, if desired.

***Makes 6 servings***

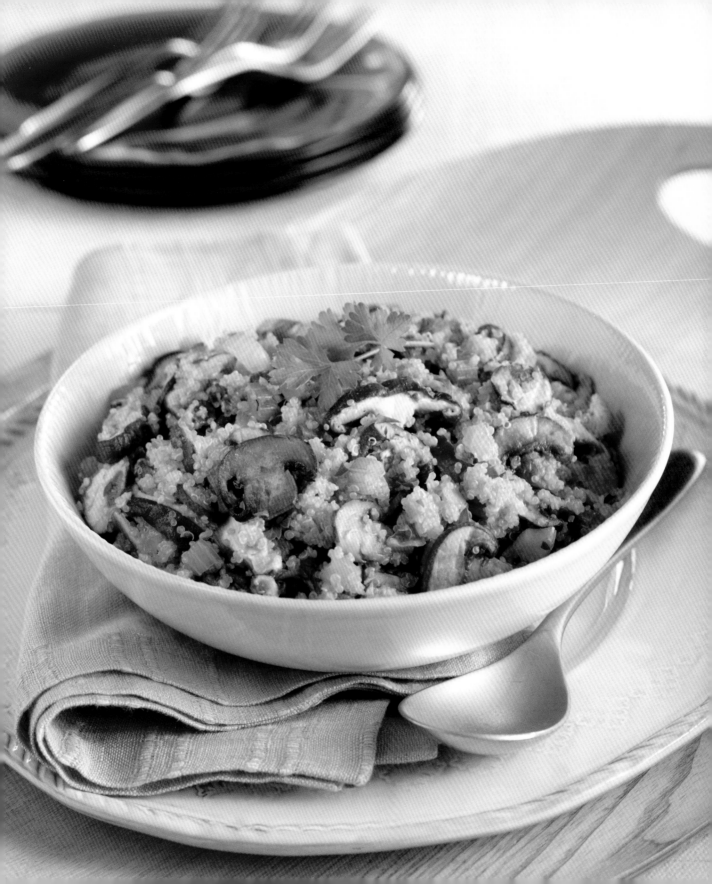

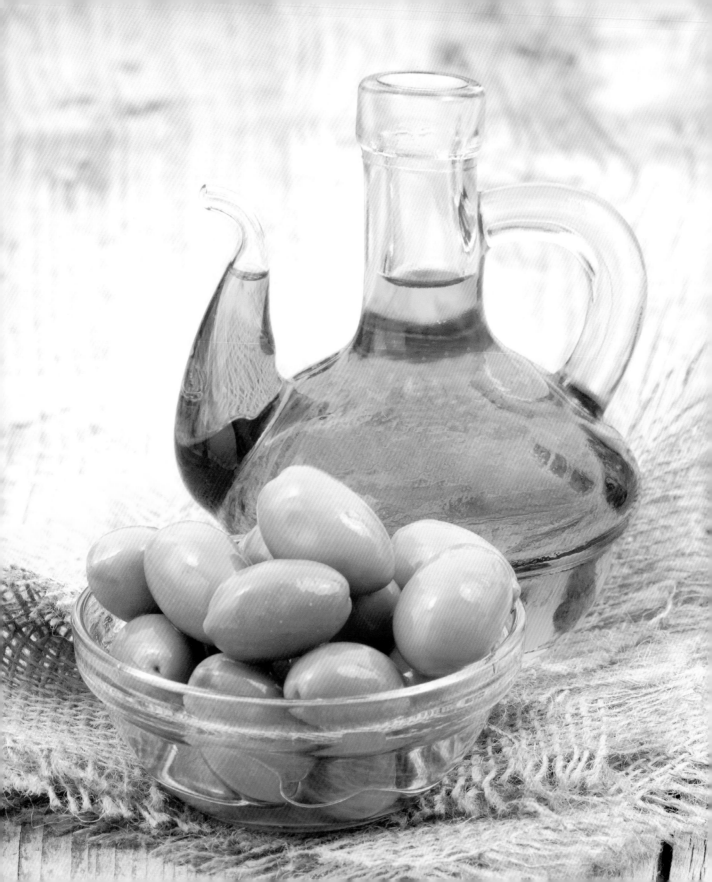

# OLIVE OIL

A key ingredient in the Mediterranean diet, olive oil adds delicious flavor to foods while providing myriad health benefits.

Olive oil is considered healthy because it's very low in the saturated fats that tend to raise levels of LDL cholesterol, and it is high in monounsaturated fats. Substituting monounsaturated fats for saturated fats has been shown to not only lower LDL but also help raise HDL cholesterol. Extra virgin and virgin olive oils are also rich in flavonoids, antioxidant phytonutrients that help protect cells from damage that can lead to heart disease and cancer. Olive oil might even play a role in controlling diabetes and weight.

# PERSIAN EGGPLANT DIP

3 large eggplants (3½ pounds total), peeled and cut into 1-inch cubes

1 teaspoon salt

5 tablespoons extra virgin olive oil, divided

2 onions, chopped

1 tablespoon dried mint

3 tablespoons plain Greek yogurt

⅓ cup finely chopped walnuts

Pita bread wedges and/or assorted vegetable sticks

**1** Toss eggplant with salt in large bowl; transfer to large colander. Place colander in large bowl or sink; let stand 1 hour at room temperature to drain.

**2** Meanwhile, heat 1 tablespoon oil in large nonstick skillet over medium-high heat. Add onions; cook 5 to 6 minutes or until lightly browned, stirring occasionally. Transfer to slow cooker. Stir in eggplant. Cover; cook on LOW 6 to 8 hours or on HIGH 3½ to 4 hours or until eggplant is very soft.

**3** Heat remaining 4 tablespoons oil in small saucepan over low heat. Add mint; cook about 15 minutes or until very fragrant. Set aside to cool slightly.

**4** Drain eggplant mixture in colander or fine-mesh strainer; press out any excess liquid with back of spoon. Return to slow cooker; mash with fork. Stir in yogurt. Sprinkle with chopped walnuts; drizzle with mint oil. Serve warm with pita bread and/or assorted vegetable sticks.

*Makes 12 to 16 servings*

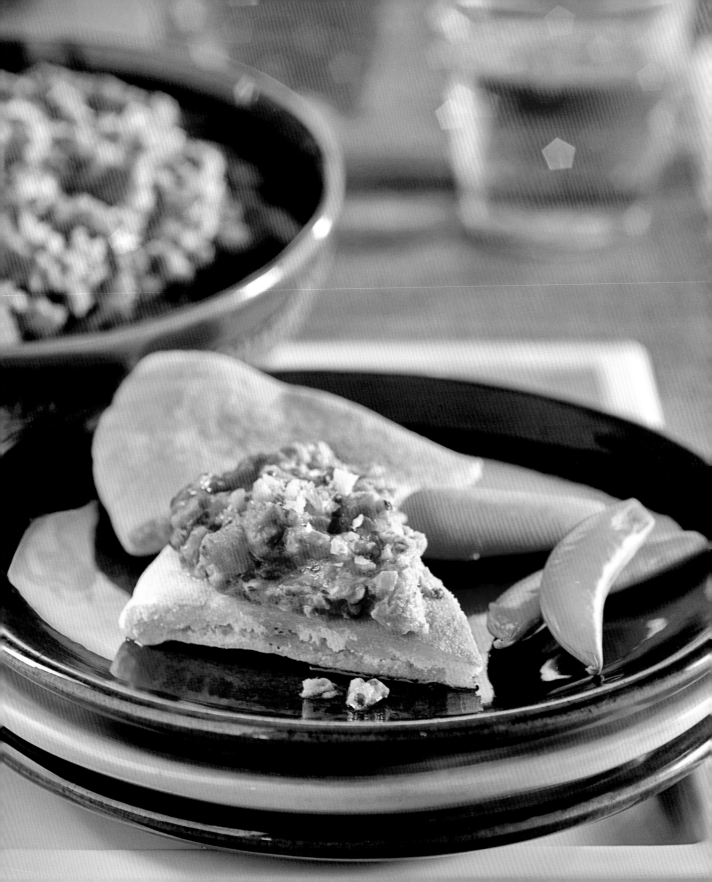

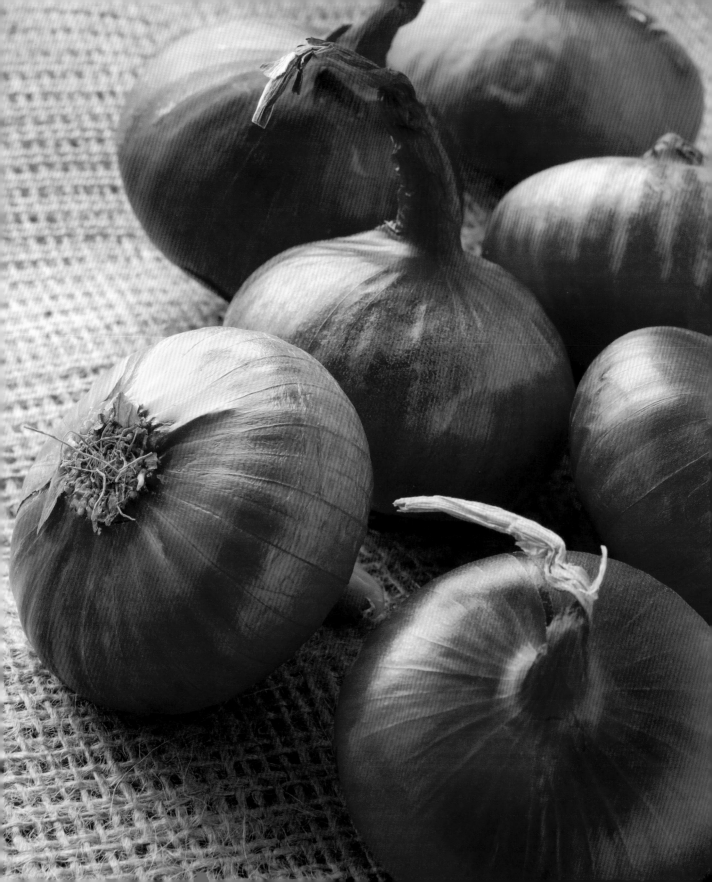

# ONIONS

Like other members of the allium family, including garlic and shallots, onions enhance the flavor of so many dishes while providing an impressive array of health benefits.

Onions contain phytonutrients that fight inflammation, which a growing body of evidence suggests may contribute to a host of chronic diseases, from cancer and heart disease to arthritis, asthma and diabetes. Onions help lower blood cholesterol and reduce blood clotting, which together can help prevent the narrowing and eventual blockage of arteries that causes heart attacks and strokes. Onions also contain vitamin C, folate and fiber. The bright green tops of green onions provide vitamin A, which is essential for skin and eye health.

# BALSAMIC BEEF, MUSHROOMS AND ONIONS

2 tablespoons olive oil, divided

2 large sweet onions, sliced

½ teaspoon salt, divided

5 teaspoons balsamic vinegar, divided

1 cup sliced mushrooms

1 boneless beef top sirloin (about 1 pound), cut into ½-inch-thick slices

¼ teaspoon dried thyme

¼ to ½ teaspoon black pepper

1 Heat 1 tablespoon oil in large skillet over medium heat. Add onions; cook and stir 15 minutes.

2 Stir in ¼ teaspoon salt. Add 3 teaspoons vinegar, 1 teaspoon at a time, stirring to scrape up any browned bits in bottom of skillet.

3 Add mushrooms; cook and stir over medium-low heat 5 minutes or until mushrooms are tender. Transfer to medium bowl; cover to keep warm.

4 Add remaining 1 tablespoon oil to skillet; heat over medium-high heat. Add beef; sprinkle with remaining ¼ teaspoon salt, thyme and pepper. Cook 4 to 6 minutes or until browned.

5 Turn off heat; drizzle with remaining 2 teaspoons balsamic vinegar Stir in vegetables. Serve immediately.

*Makes 4 servings*

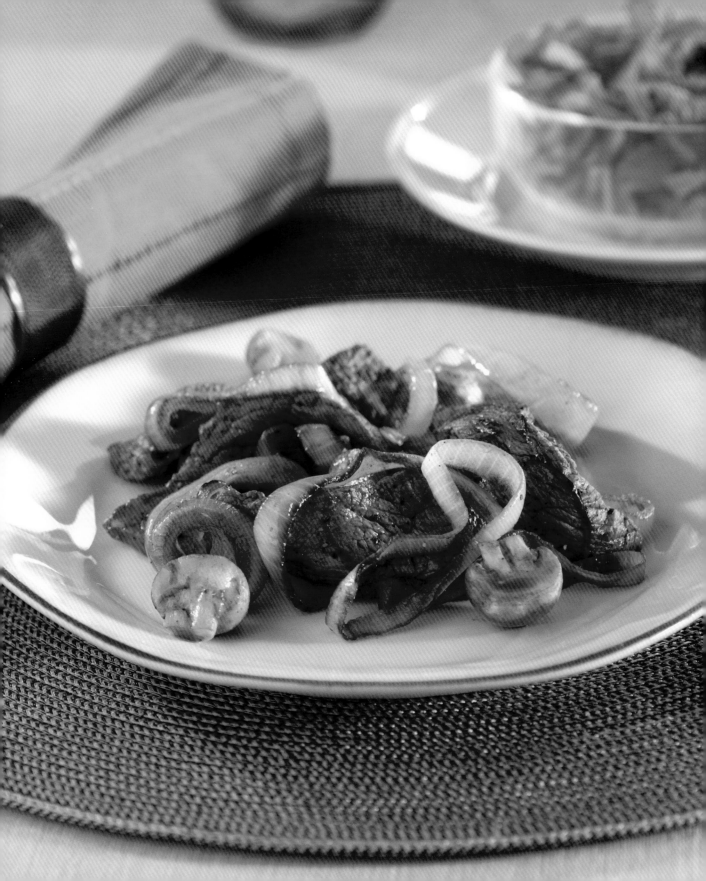

# ORANGE CHICKEN STIR-FRY over QUINOA

½ cup uncooked quinoa

1 cup water

2 teaspoons coconut oil, divided

1 pound boneless skinless chicken breasts, cut into thin strips

1 cup fresh orange juice (2 to 3 oranges)

1 tablespoon reduced-sodium soy sauce

1 tablespoon cornstarch

½ cup sliced green onions

2 tablespoons grated fresh ginger

6 ounces snow peas, ends trimmed

1 cup thinly sliced carrots

¼ teaspoon red pepper flakes (optional)

1 Place quinoa in fine-mesh strainer; rinse well under cold running water. Bring 1 cup water to a boil in medium saucepan over high heat; stir in quinoa. Reduce heat to low; cover and simmer 10 to 15 minutes or until quinoa is tender and water is absorbed.

2 Meanwhile, heat 1 teaspoon oil in large skillet over medium-high heat. Add chicken; cook and stir 4 to 6 minutes or until no longer pink. Remove to plate; keep warm.

3 Stir orange juice and soy sauce into cornstarch in small bowl until smooth; set aside.

4 Heat remaining 1 teaspoon oil in skillet. Add green onions and ginger; stir-fry 2 minutes. Add snow peas and carrots; stir-fry 4 to 5 minutes or until carrots are crisp-tender.

5 Return chicken to skillet. Stir orange juice mixture; add to skillet and bring to a boil. Reduce heat to low; cook until sauce is slightly thickened. Serve chicken and vegetables over quinoa; sprinkle with red pepper flakes, if desired.

*Makes 4 servings*

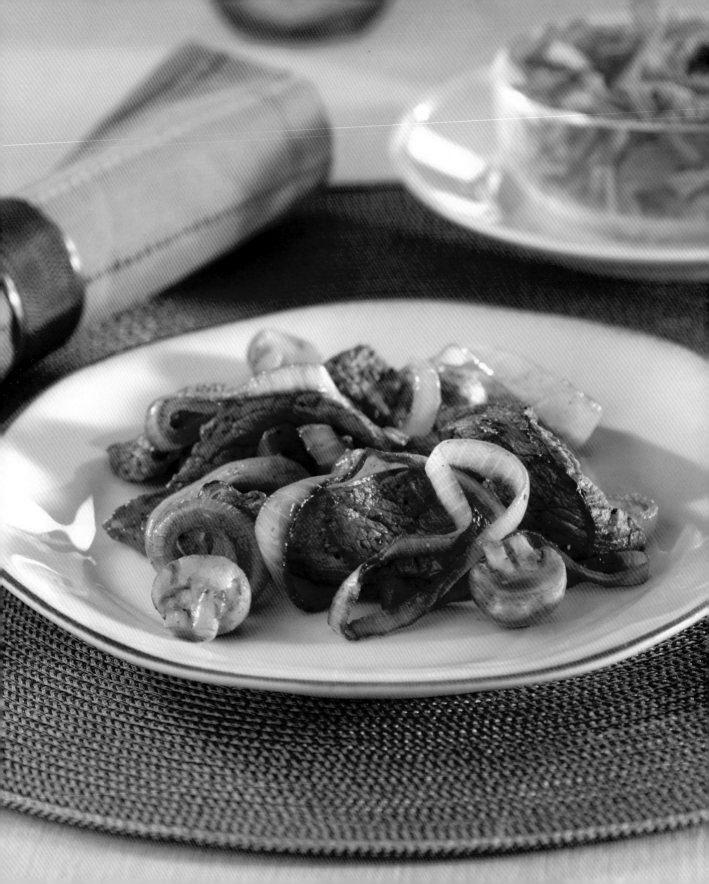

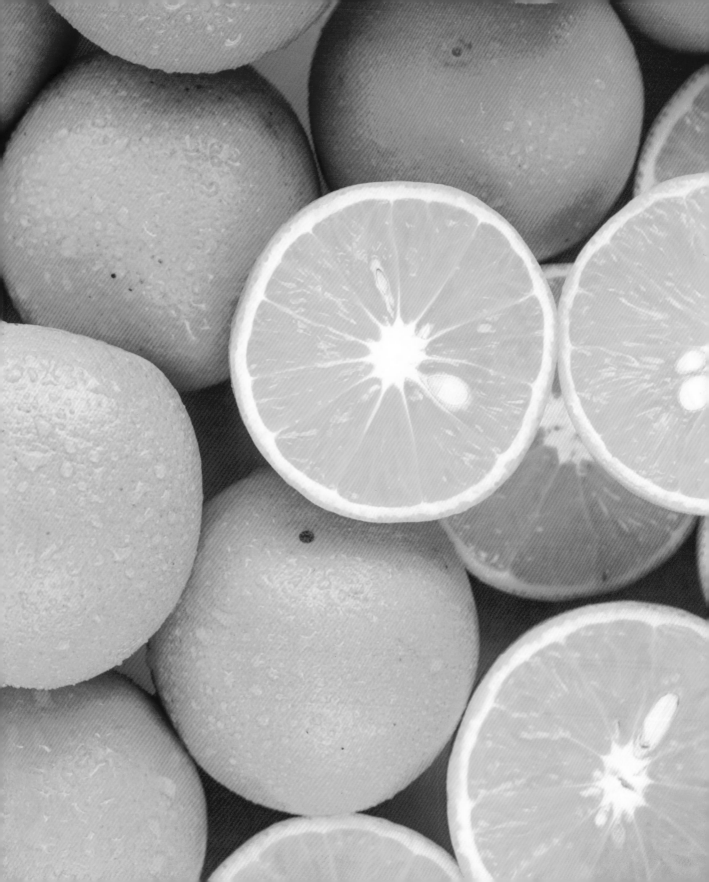

# ORANGES

Oranges are best known for their abundant vitamin C—one orange provides 130 percent of the daily requirement for this antioxidant vitamin, which helps protect the heart and eyes, ward off infections, heal wounds, and maintain healthy teeth, gums, skin, bones and blood vessels.

But oranges also contain potassium for healthy blood pressure, folate to prevent certain birth defects, and soluble fiber to help with blood sugar control. And an array of phytonutrients, some concentrated in the skin and pulp of the orange, offer protection from a host of common diseases and health problems.

# ORANGE CHICKEN STIR-FRY over QUINOA

½ cup uncooked quinoa

1 cup water

2 teaspoons coconut oil, divided

1 pound boneless skinless chicken breasts, cut into thin strips

1 cup fresh orange juice (2 to 3 oranges)

1 tablespoon reduced-sodium soy sauce

1 tablespoon cornstarch

½ cup sliced green onions

2 tablespoons grated fresh ginger

6 ounces snow peas, ends trimmed

1 cup thinly sliced carrots

¼ teaspoon red pepper flakes (optional)

1 Place quinoa in fine-mesh strainer; rinse well under cold running water. Bring 1 cup water to a boil in medium saucepan over high heat; stir in quinoa. Reduce heat to low; cover and simmer 10 to 15 minutes or until quinoa is tender and water is absorbed.

2 Meanwhile, heat 1 teaspoon oil in large skillet over medium-high heat. Add chicken; cook and stir 4 to 6 minutes or until no longer pink. Remove to plate; keep warm.

3 Stir orange juice and soy sauce into cornstarch in small bowl until smooth; set aside.

4 Heat remaining 1 teaspoon oil in skillet. Add green onions and ginger; stir-fry 2 minutes. Add snow peas and carrots; stir-fry 4 to 5 minutes or until carrots are crisp-tender.

5 Return chicken to skillet. Stir orange juice mixture; add to skillet and bring to a boil. Reduce heat to low; cook until sauce is slightly thickened. Serve chicken and vegetables over quinoa; sprinkle with red pepper flakes, if desired.

*Makes 4 servings*

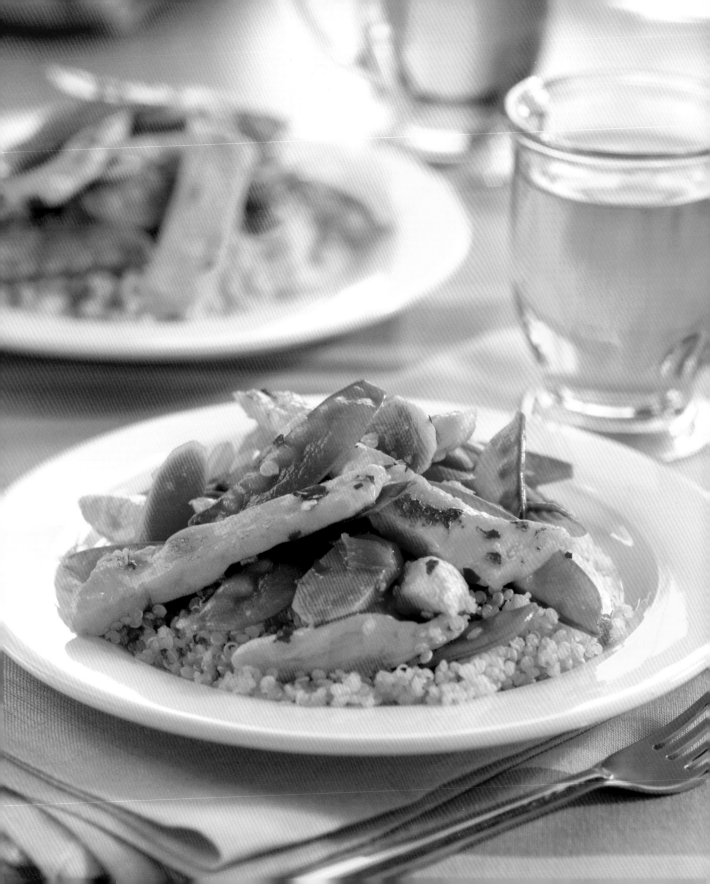

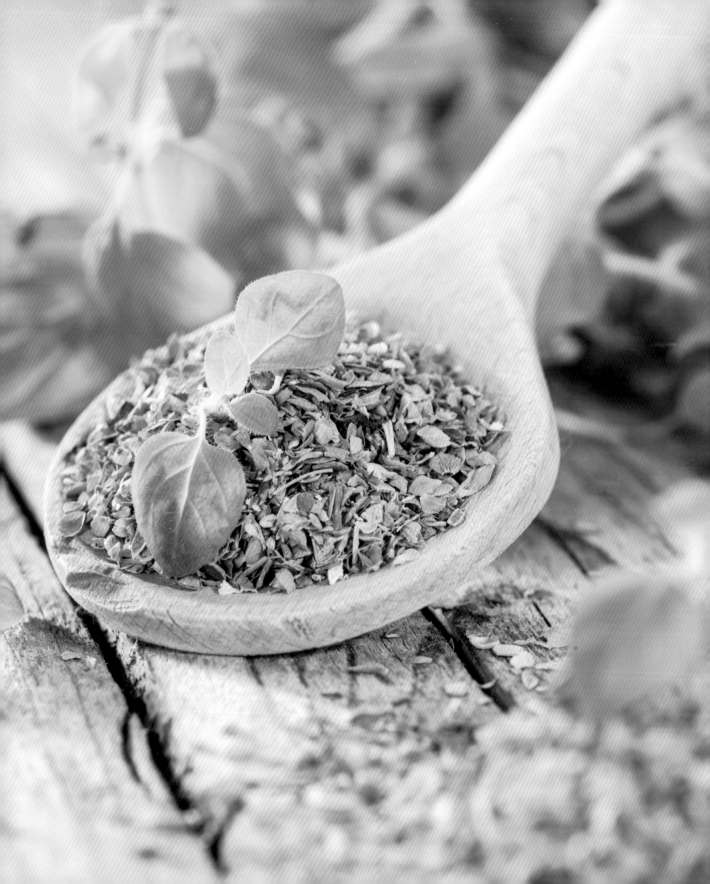

# OREGANO

In ancient times oregano was prescribed for many ailments and was also considered a good luck charm—seemingly with good reason. Oregano has one of the highest antioxidant levels of all herbs—just one teaspoon of dried oregano has more antioxidants than a serving of almonds or asparagus.

Whether fresh or dried, oregano is bursting with potent antioxidant nutrients that give it serious disease-fighting potential. The specific medicinal effects associated with oregano are still being researched but may include preventing the growth of cancerous cells and fighting the growth of bacteria and parasites that can cause ulcers and other gastrointestinal problems. Oregano is also a good source of lutein and zeaxanthin, phytonutrients that help cataracts and certain other eye diseases.

# GREEK SALAD BOWL

1 cup uncooked pearled farro

2½ cups water

1¼ teaspoons dried oregano, divided

½ teaspoon salt, divided

¼ cup extra virgin olive oil

2 tablespoons red wine vinegar

1 clove garlic, minced

⅛ teaspoon black pepper

2 cucumbers, julienned, cubed or thinly sliced

½ red onion, thinly sliced

2 medium tomatoes, diced

1 can (about 15 ounces) chickpeas, rinsed and drained

4 ounces feta cheese, cubed or crumbled

1 Rinse farro under cold running water; place in medium saucepan. Add 2½ cups water, 1 teaspoon oregano and ¼ teaspoon salt; bring to a boil over high heat. Reduce heat to medium-low; cook 20 minutes or until farro is tender. Drain any remaining water.

2 Whisk oil, vinegar, garlic, remaining ¼ teaspoon salt, ¼ teaspoon oregano and pepper in small bowl until well blended.

3 Divide farro among four bowls; top with cucumbers, onion, tomatoes, chickpeas and cheese. Drizzle with dressing.

*Makes 4 servings*

**VARIATION:** Add grilled chicken or lamb for a heartier meal, or stir all ingredients together and serve as a side dish.

**NOTE:** This is a great recipe to use a spiralizer if you have one. Cut the ends off the cucumbers and spiral with the thin ribbon blade. Spiral the red onion with the thin ribbon blade and chop into shorter lengths.

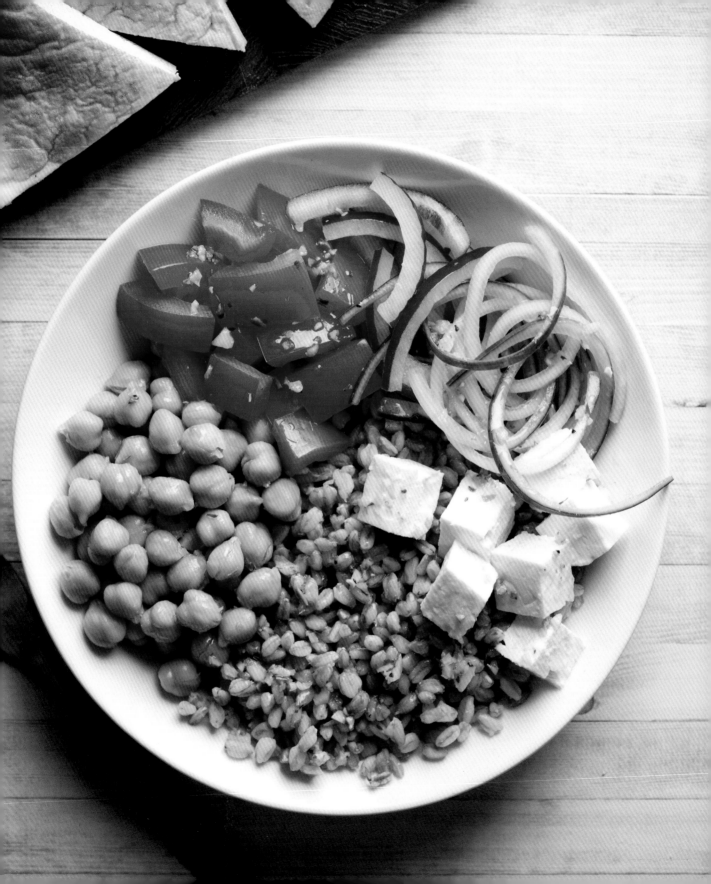

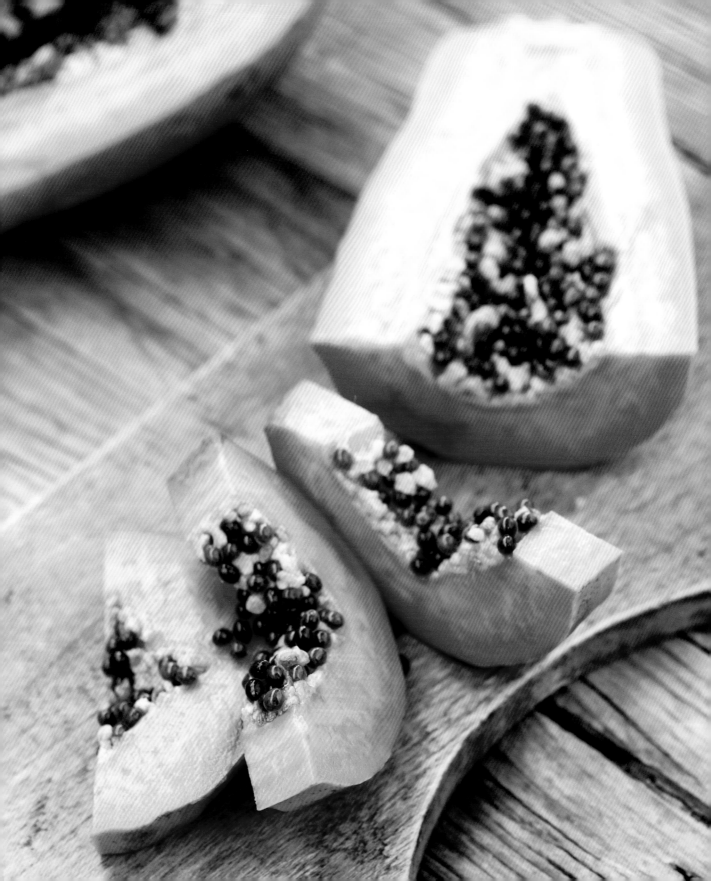

# PAPAYA

With its golden skin and shiny black seeds, tropical papaya is an amazing fruit that can weigh up to 20 pounds.

Used both green and ripe, this sweet and tart fruit is bursting with vitamins A and C, antioxidants that help reduce heart disease and cancer risks. The generous dose of vitamin C also fortifies your body's wound-healing ability and helps keep your immune system in good shape, so it can protect your body from unhealthy invaders. In addition, papayas provide plenty of potassium, an essential mineral that helps control blood pressure, and folate, a B vitamin needed during pregnancy to reduce the risk of birth defects. The fiber in papayas is mostly soluble, so it helps lower blood cholesterol.

# HOT AND SPICY FRUIT SALAD

⅓ cup orange juice

3 tablespoons lime juice

3 tablespoons minced fresh mint, basil or cilantro

2 jalapeño peppers,* seeded and minced

1 tablespoon honey

½ small honeydew melon, cut into cubes

1 ripe large papaya, peeled, seeded and cubed

1 pint fresh strawberries, stemmed and halved

1 can (8 ounces) pineapple chunks, drained

*Jalapeño peppers can sting and irritate the skin, so wear rubber gloves when handling peppers and do not touch your eyes.

1 Whisk orange juice, lime juice, mint, jalapeño peppers and honey in small bowl until well blended.

2 Combine melon, papaya, strawberries and pineapple in large bowl. Pour orange juice mixture over fruit; toss gently to coat.

3 Serve immediately or cover and refrigerate up to 3 hours.

*Makes 6 servings*

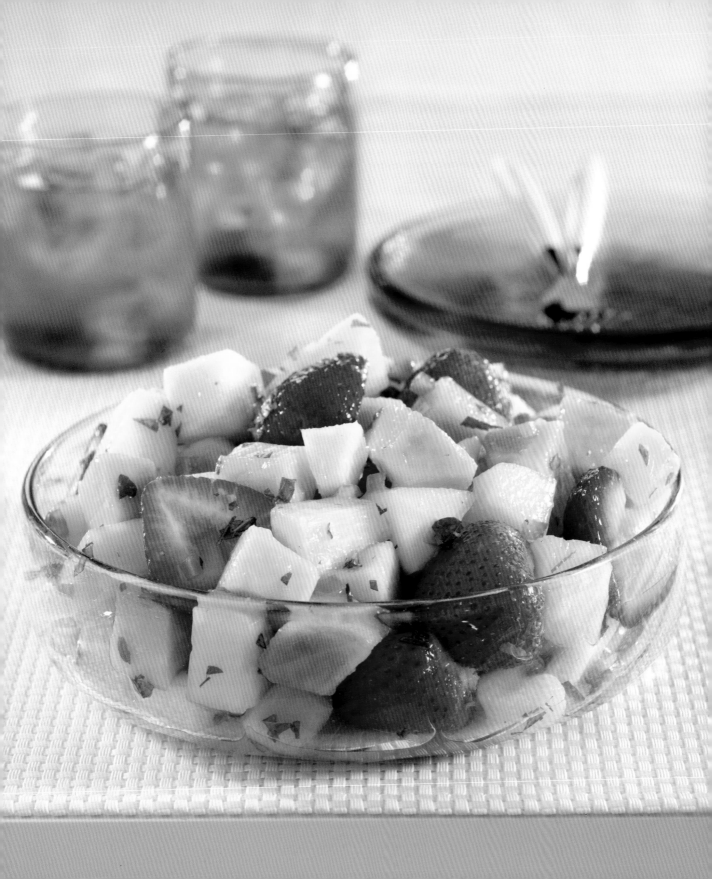

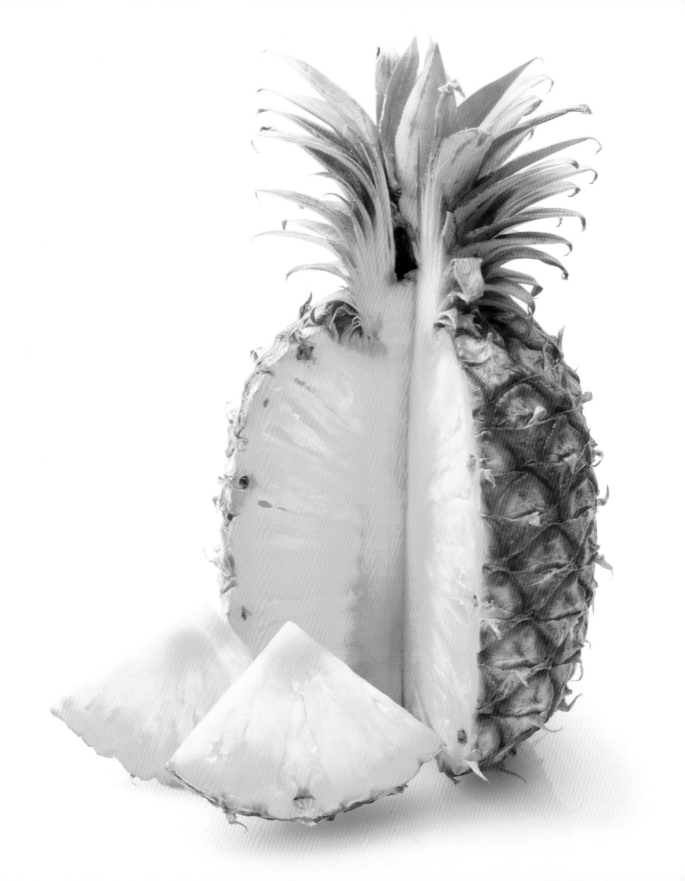

# PINEAPPLE

Pineapple is much loved for its unique sweet and tart taste; it is also high in fiber and other health benefits.

Pineapple is simply packed with nutrients—just ½ cup offers more than a third of your daily requirement for vitamin C, which helps keep your immune system in good condition to resist colds, flu and other infectious diseases. One cup provides more than the recommended daily intake of manganese, a mineral essential for energy production and strong bones. This tropical treat also provides copper, needed for proper brain and nerve function, and folate for preventing certain birth defects. Fresh raw pineapple contains the enzyme bromelain, a digestive aid that also helps prevent inflammation and swelling.

# SPICED SALMON WITH PINEAPPLE-GINGER SALSA

## SALMON

- 1 **teaspoon ground cumin**
- ½ **teaspoon ground allspice**
- ¼ **teaspoon salt**
- ¼ **teaspoon black pepper**
- 4 **salmon steaks (4 ounces each), rinsed and patted dry**

## SALSA

- ¾ **cup finely chopped fresh pineapple**
- ¼ **cup finely chopped poblano pepper**
- 2 **tablespoons chopped fresh cilantro**
- 1 **tablespoon lime juice**
- 1 **teaspoon honey**
- 1 **teaspoon grated fresh ginger**
- ½ **teaspoon grated orange peel**

**1** Preheat oven to 350°F. Line baking sheet with foil; spray with nonstick cooking spray.

**2** Combine cumin, allspice, salt and black pepper in small bowl; mix well. Sprinkle over both sides of salmon, pressing lightly to adhere. Place salmon on prepared baking sheet.

**3** Bake 14 to 16 minutes or until fish is opaque in center.

**4** Meanwhile, combine pineapple, poblano pepper, cilantro, lime juice, honey, ginger and orange peel in small bowl; mix well. Serve over salmon.

*Makes 4 servings*

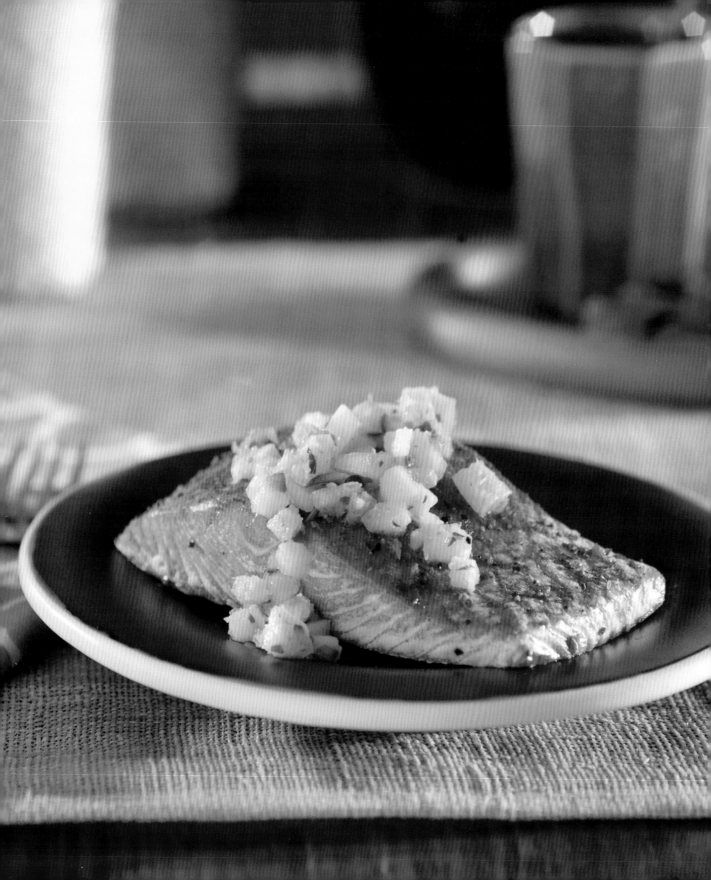

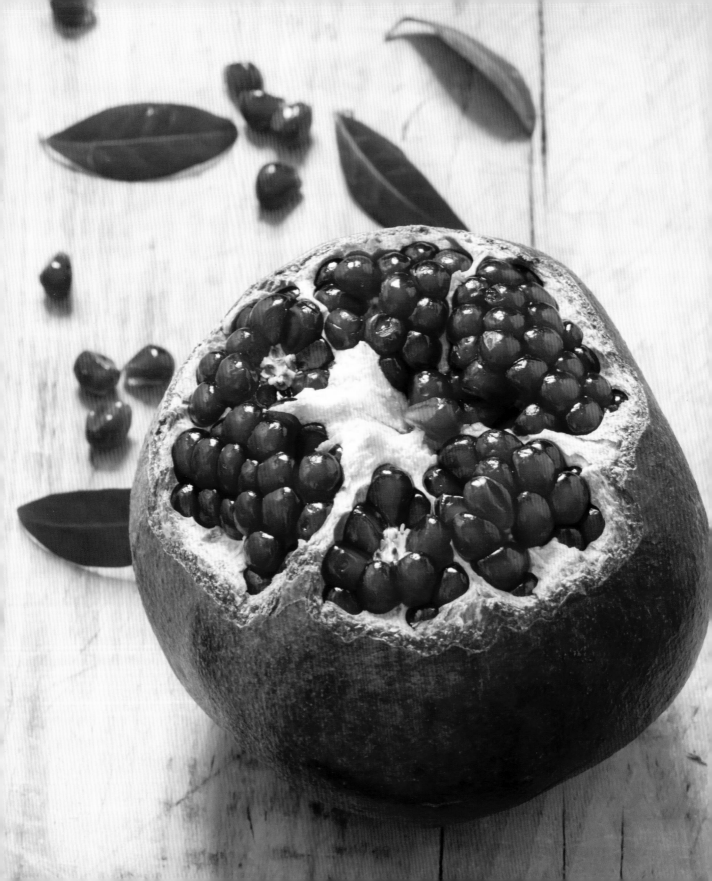

# POMEGRANATES

Pomegranates may require extra effort to eat, but they are worth the effort—those sparkling little seeds and their juice are loaded with nutrients.

Pomegranates offer up plenty of potassium, a mineral that plays an important role in balancing fluids in the body and controlling blood pressure. The seeds (arils) contain plenty of fiber that helps keep you regular, while the juice is rich in disease-fighting antioxidants, with close to three times the antioxidants as green tea or red wine. Pomegranate juice may help reduce the buildup of artery-clogging plaque, lower levels of LDL ("bad") cholesterol, and help improve blood flow.

# SPINACH SALAD WITH POMEGRANATE VINAIGRETTE

1 package (5 ounces) baby spinach

½ cup pomegranate seeds (arils)

¼ cup crumbled goat cheese

2 tablespoons chopped walnuts, toasted*

¼ cup pomegranate juice

2 tablespoons extra virgin olive oil

1 tablespoon honey

1 tablespoon red wine vinegar

¼ teaspoon salt

¼ teaspoon black pepper

*To toast walnuts, cook in small skillet over medium heat 1 to 2 minutes or until nuts are lightly browned, stirring frequently.*

1 Combine spinach, pomegranate seeds, goat cheese and walnuts in large bowl.

2 Whisk pomegranate juice, oil, honey, vinegar, salt and pepper in small bowl until well blended. Pour over salad; toss gently to coat. Serve immediately.

*Makes 4 servings*

**TIP:** For easier removal of pomegranate seeds, cut a pomegranate into pieces and immerse in a bowl of cold water. The membrane that holds the seeds in place will float to the top; discard it and collect the seeds. For convenience, you can find containers of ready-to-use pomegranate seeds in the refrigerated produce section of some supermarkets.

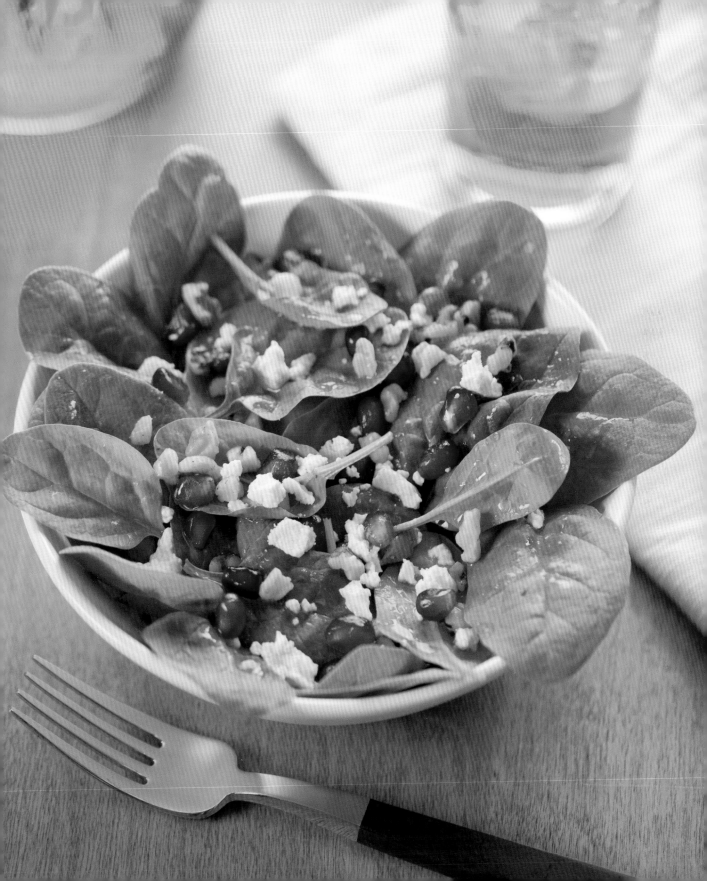

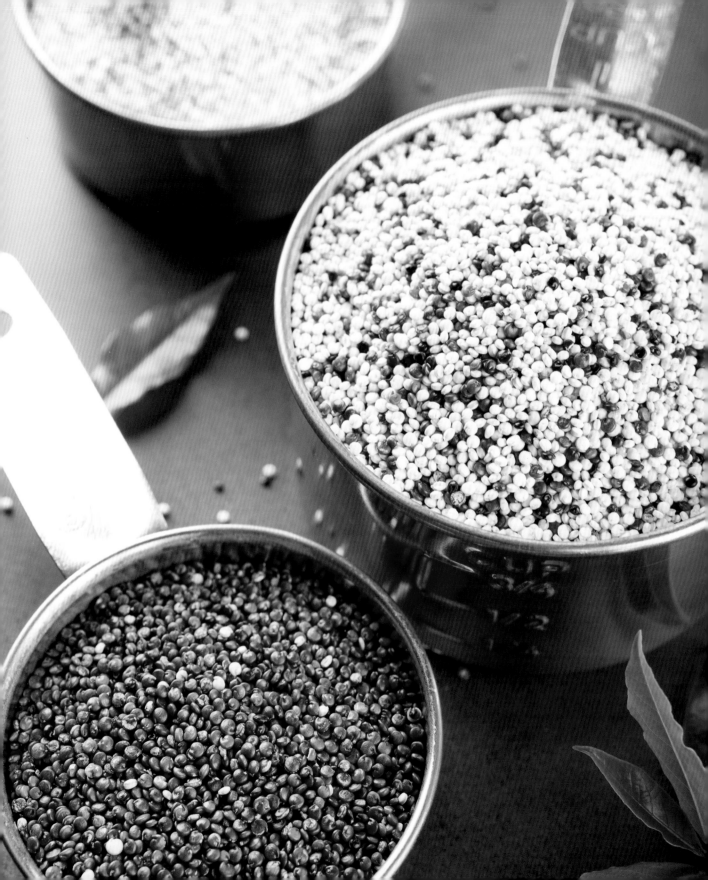

# QUINOA

This newly popular ancient grain is truly amazing—it provides a rich and balanced source of vital nutrients and more protein than any other grain.

Quinoa is a unique grain because its protein is considered complete; it provides all of the essential amino acids, while other grains are missing the essential amino acid called lysine. It is also higher in unsaturated fats and lower in carbohydrates than most other grains. It is an excellent source of numerous minerals, including iron, magnesium, potassium, phosphorus and zinc, and it also provides fiber, making it an all-around healthy grain. In addition, quinoa contains phytonutrients called saponins, which have anticancer and anti-inflammatory properties and may inhibit cholesterol absorption.

# QUINOA BURRITO BOWLS

1 cup uncooked quinoa

2 cups water

2 tablespoons lime juice, divided

1 tablespoon olive oil

1 small onion, diced

1 red bell pepper, diced

1 clove garlic, minced

½ cup canned black beans, rinsed and drained

½ cup thawed frozen corn

¼ teaspoon salt

¼ cup Greek yogurt or light sour cream

Shredded lettuce

Lime wedges (optional)

1 Place quinoa in fine-mesh strainer; rinse well under cold running water. Bring 2 cups water to a boil in small saucepan over high heat; stir in quinoa. Reduce heat to low; cover and simmer 10 to 15 minutes or until quinoa is tender and water is absorbed. Stir in 1 tablespoon lime juice. Cover and keep warm.

2 Meanwhile, heat oil in large skillet over medium heat. Add onion and bell pepper; cook and stir 5 minutes or until vegetables are tender. Add garlic; cook and stir 1 minute. Add black beans, corn and salt; cook 5 minutes or until heated through.

3 Combine yogurt and remaining 1 tablespoon lime juice in small bowl; mix well.

4 Divide quinoa among four serving bowls; top with black bean mixture, lettuce and yogurt mixture. Garnish with lime wedges.

*Makes 4 servings*

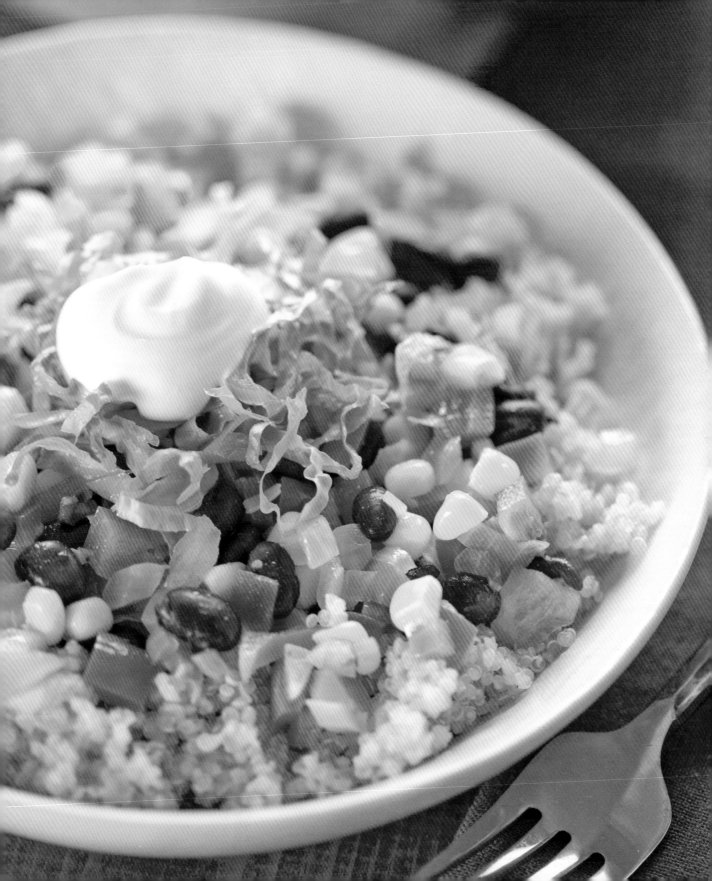

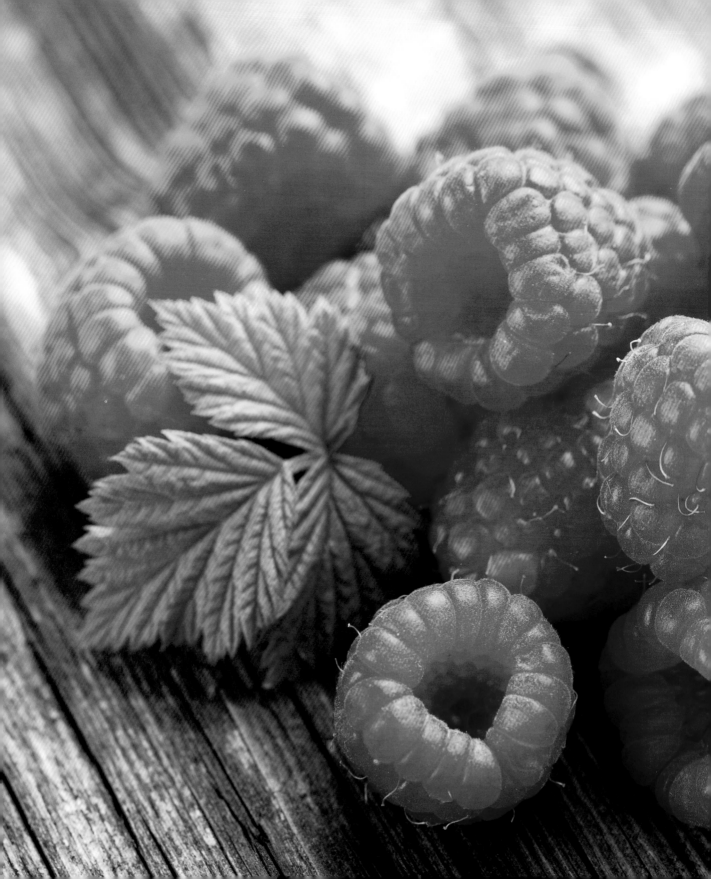

# RASPBERRIES

Raspberries are a member of the rose family; while they may appear fragile and delicate, they actually pack a powerful nutritional punch.

Raspberries provide a whopping 8 grams of fiber per cup, fitting in well with a high-fiber diet which is associated with a lower risk of chronic diseases. Raspberries are high in pectin, a form of soluble fiber known to help lower blood cholesterol; the insoluble fiber in raspberry seeds helps prevent and treat constipation and other digestive woes. Raspberries are also a good source of vitamin C, an antioxidant, and ellagic acid, a phytochemical, both of which help fight against cancer.

# CREAMY RASPBERRY SMOOTHIE

1   cup almond milk

2   cups frozen raspberries

½   avocado

2   tablespoons lemon juice

Combine almond milk, raspberries, avocado and lemon juice in blender; blend until smooth.

*Makes 2 servings*

# CHOCOLATE RASPBERRY SMOOTHIE

½   cup unsweetened almond or coconut milk

1   cup frozen raspberries

1   tablespoon unsweetened cocoa powder

1   teaspoon honey

Combine almond milk, raspberries, cocoa and honey in blender; blend until smooth.

*Makes 1 serving*

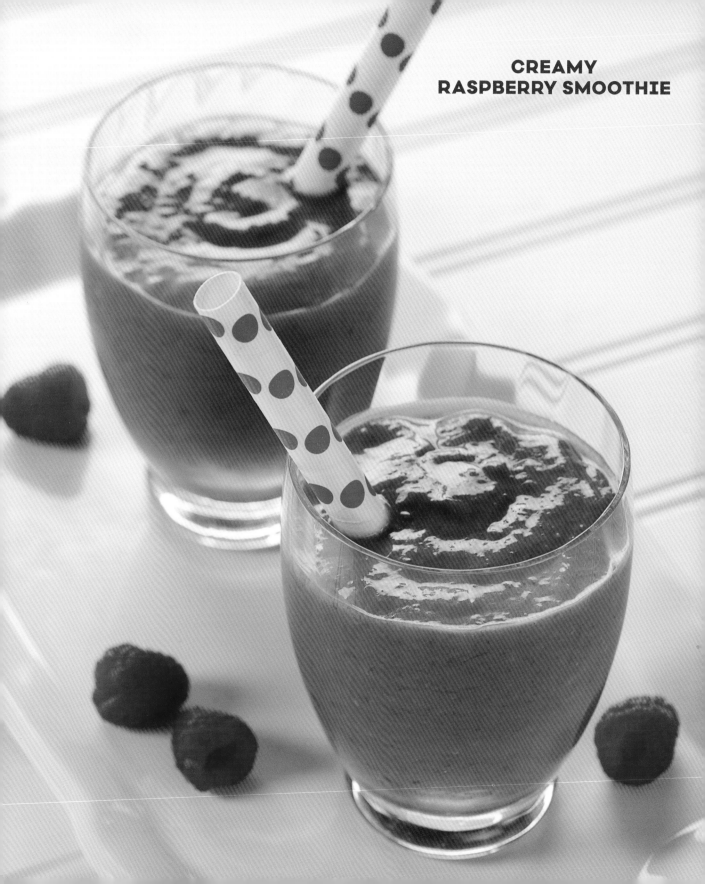

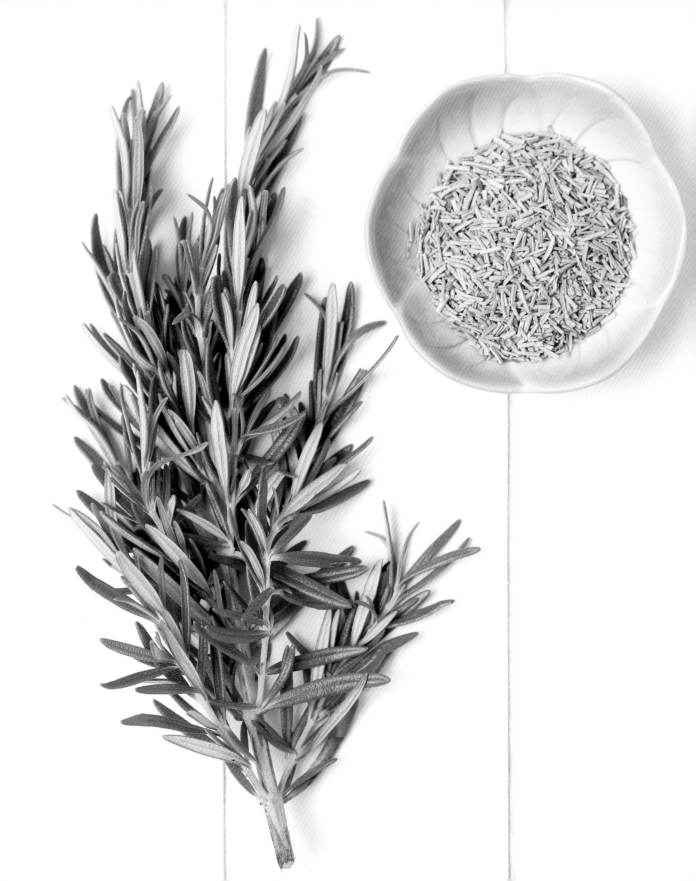

# ROSEMARY

Fragrant rosemary is a traditional culinary and apothecary herb. Although small amounts like those used in cooking are generally not considered large enough to have an effect on the body, regular use of the leaves in your food will allow you to reap the benefits of this woody herb.

Rosemary is rich in essential oils that help stimulate the immune system and improve digestion. Rosemary has been shown to be a cognitive stimulant, increasing blood flow to the head and brain and improving concentration; it also acts as a stimulant for the body and boosts the production of red blood cells and blood flow. The aroma of rosemary has been linked to improved mood and stress reduction, while the consumption of rosemary has been used by many cultures as a remedy for digestive disorders.

# LEMON ROSEMARY ROASTED CHICKEN AND POTATOES

4 bone-in skin-on chicken breasts

½ cup lemon juice

6 tablespoons olive oil, divided

6 cloves garlic, minced, divided

2 tablespoons plus 1 teaspoon chopped fresh rosemary leaves *or* 2¼ teaspoons dried rosemary, divided

1½ teaspoons salt, divided

2 pounds unpeeled small red potatoes, cut into quarters

1 large onion, cut into 2-inch pieces

¼ teaspoon black pepper

**1** Place chicken in large resealable food storage bag. Combine lemon juice, 3 tablespoons oil, 3 cloves garlic, 1 tablespoon rosemary and ½ teaspoon salt in small bowl; pour over chicken. Seal bag; turn to coat. Refrigerate several hours or overnight.

**2** Preheat oven to 400°F. Combine potatoes and onion in roasting pan. Combine remaining 3 tablespoons oil, 3 cloves garlic, 1 tablespoon rosemary, 1 teaspoon salt and pepper in small bowl; mix well. Pour over vegetables; toss to coat.

**3** Drain chicken; discard marinade. Arrange chicken in pan with vegetables in single layer; sprinkle with remaining 1 teaspoon rosemary.

**4** Roast about 50 minutes or until potatoes are tender and chicken is cooked through (165°F). Sprinkle with additional salt and pepper to taste.

*Makes 4 servings*

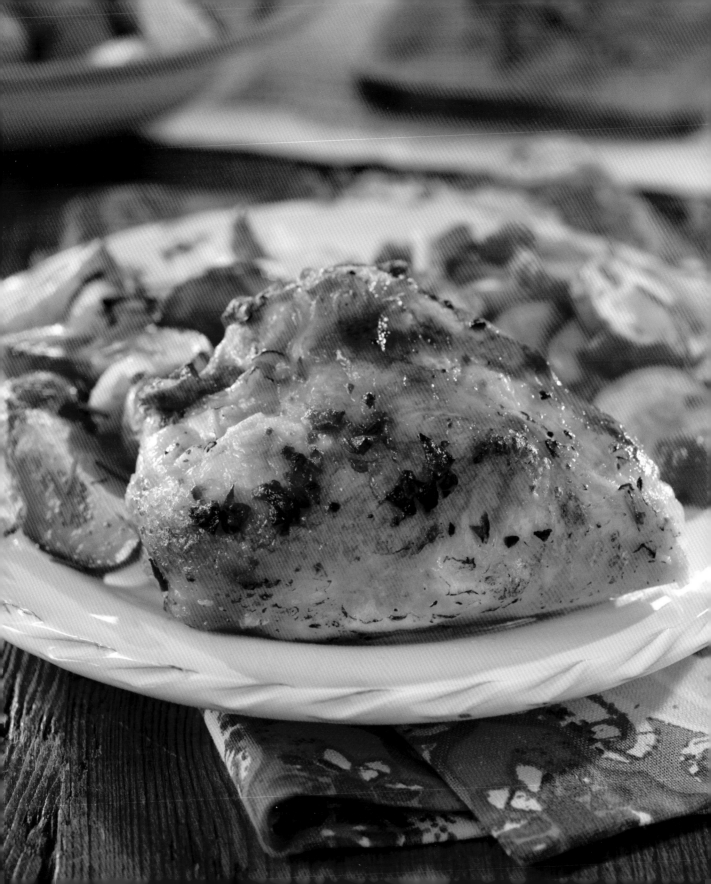

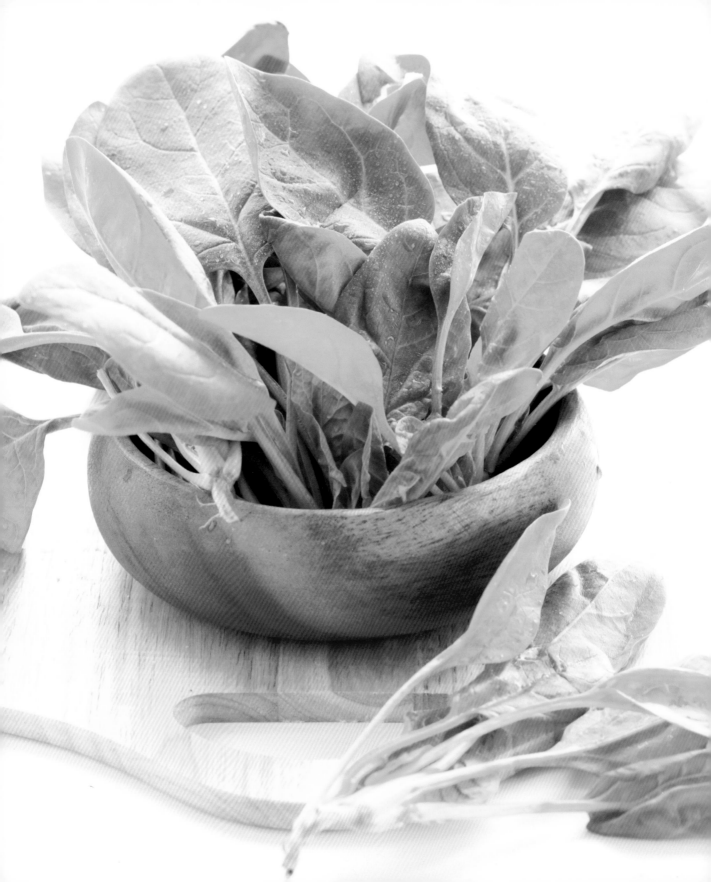

# SPINACH

Spinach is a nutritional superstar, loaded with vitamins and minerals and offering twice as much fiber as most other cooking and salad greens.

Like other dark greens, spinach contains an amazingly rich mix of essential nutrients with antioxidant functions, including vitamins C, E and A and the minerals manganese, selenium and zinc. Spinach also provides more than a dozen antioxidant and anti-inflammatory phytonutrients—this makes spinach helpful in fighting high blood pressure, hardening of the arteries, heart disease and stroke; various cancers, including those of the stomach, skin, prostate and breast; and eye diseases such as cataracts and macular degeneration. Spinach also contributes iron and folic acid for healthy red blood cells.

# FARRO, CHICKPEA AND SPINACH SALAD

4 cups water

1 cup uncooked pearled farro

3 cups baby spinach

1 medium cucumber, chopped

1 can (about 15 ounces) chickpeas, rinsed and drained

¾ cup pitted kalamata olives

¼ cup extra virgin olive oil

3 tablespoons white or golden balsamic vinegar

1 teaspoon chopped fresh rosemary leaves

1 teaspoon salt

1 clove garlic, minced

⅛ to ¼ teaspoon red pepper flakes (optional)

½ cup crumbled goat or feta cheese

**1** Bring 4 cups water to a boil in medium saucepan over high heat. Stir in farro. Reduce heat to medium-low; cook 20 to 25 minutes or until farro is tender. Drain and rinse under cold running water until cool.

**2** Combine spinach, cucumber, chickpeas, olives, oil, vinegar, rosemary, salt, garlic and red pepper flakes, if desired, in large bowl; mix well.

**3** Add farro to salad; stir until blended. Gently stir in cheese.

*Makes 4 to 6 main-dish servings*

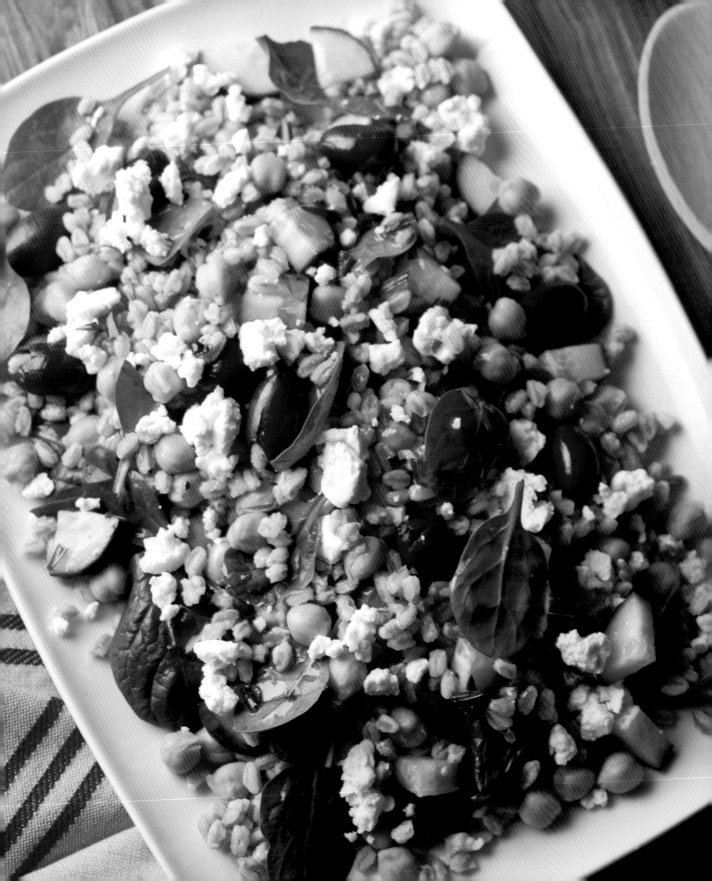

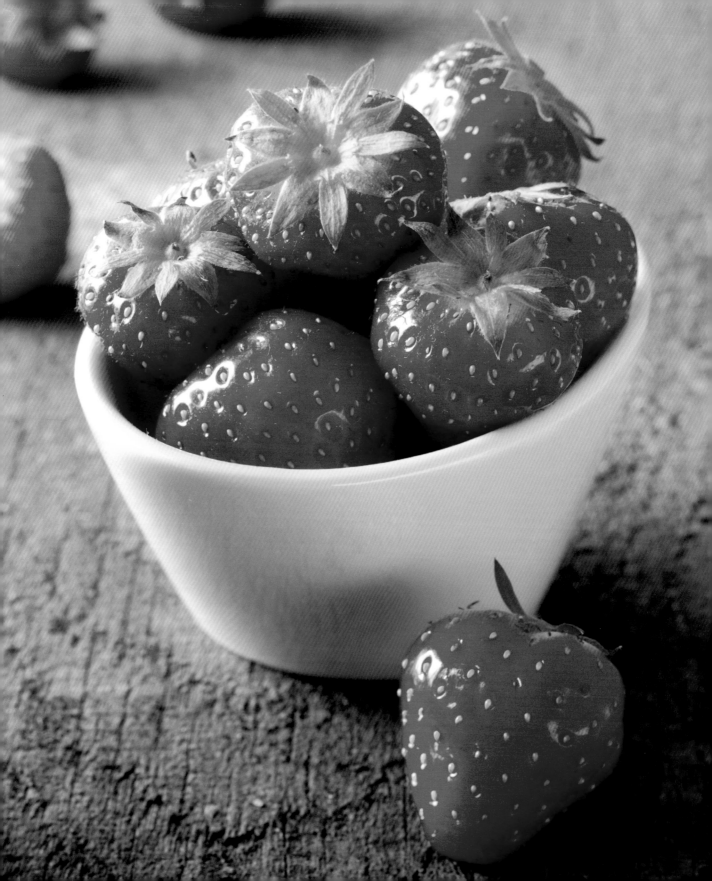

# STRAWBERRIES

Like other berries, sweet juicy strawberries pack an incredible amount of nutrients into a very small package.

Strawberries are the only fruit with seeds on the outside rather than on the inside, and these little seeds are loaded with insoluble fiber that helps keeps you regular and fend off digestive system woes, including hemorrhoids and constipation. Strawberries are a super source of disease-fighting, immunity-boosting vitamin C—even better than oranges and grapefruit. Strawberries pack plenty of potassium, an essential mineral that helps the body maintain a healthy blood pressure and so may help prevent strokes. Strawberries also contain ellagic acid, a phytonutrient with cancer-fighting and anti-inflammatory power.

# FRESH SPINACH-STRAWBERRY SALAD

- 2 to 4 ounces slivered almonds
- 1 package (9 ounces) fresh spinach
- 3 ounces thinly sliced red onion (¾ cup)
- ⅓ cup pomegranate juice
- 2 tablespoons honey
- 3 tablespoons cider vinegar
- 2 tablespoons safflower oil
- 2 tablespoons dark sesame oil
- 1 teaspoon grated fresh ginger
- ¼ teaspoon salt
- ¼ teaspoon red pepper flakes
- 2 cups quartered hulled fresh strawberries
- 4 ounces goat cheese, crumbled

**1** Cook and stir almonds in medium skillet over medium heat 2 minutes or until nuts begin to brown. Transfer to plate; set aside to cool.

**2** Combine spinach and onion in large bowl. Combine pomegranate juice, honey, vinegar, safflower oil, sesame oil, ginger, salt and red pepper flakes in small jar; cover and shake until well blended.

**3** Pour dressing over spinach and onion; toss to coat. Add strawberries; toss gently. Top with almonds and cheese. Serve immediately.

*Makes 4 to 6 servings*

**NOTE:** The dressing may be prepared up to 2 days in advance and refrigerated. Shake well before using; toss with spinach just before serving.

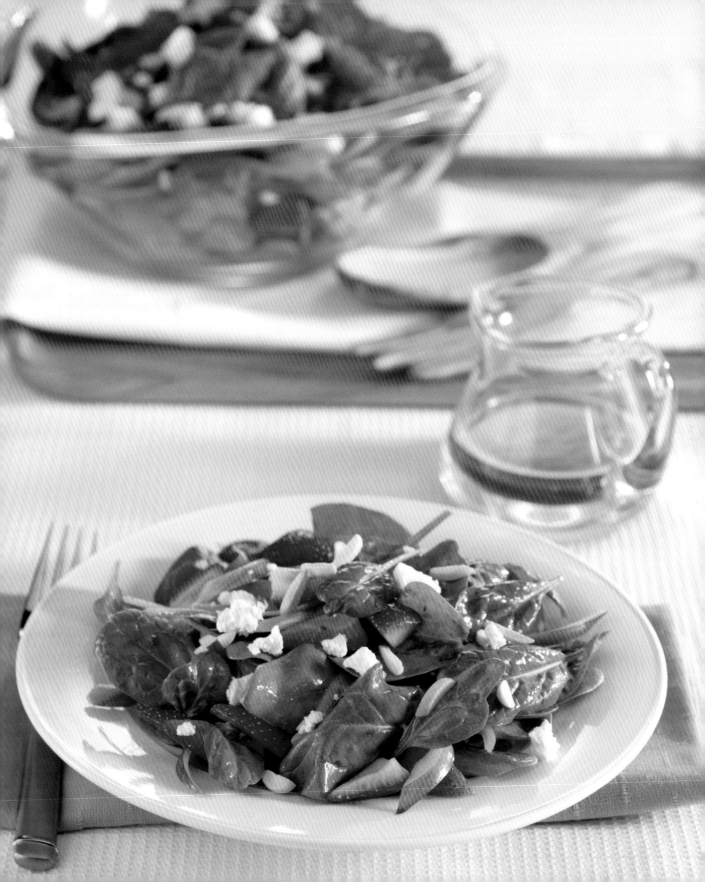

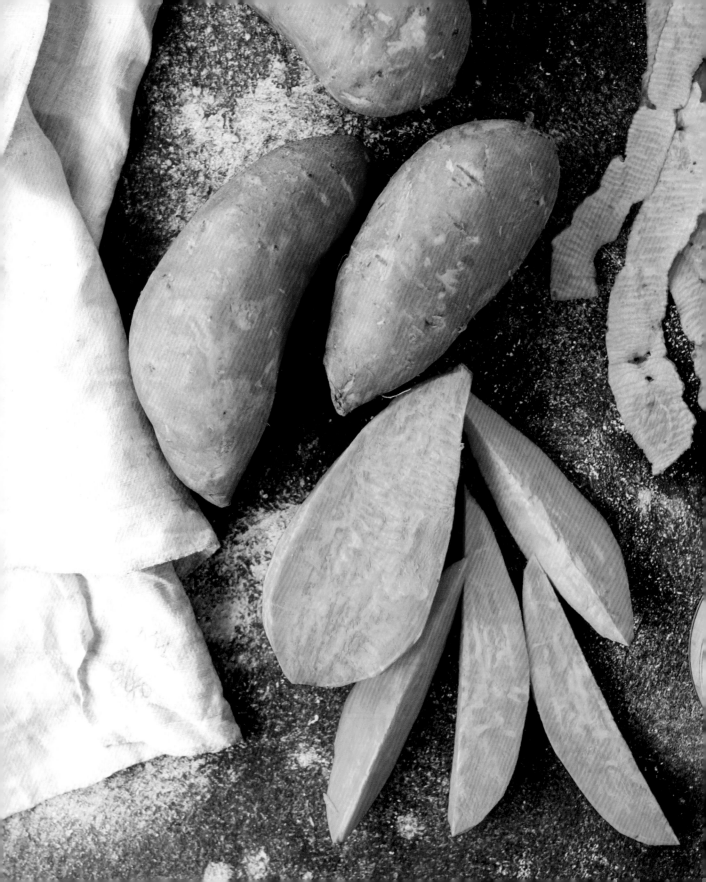

# SWEET POTATOES

These tasty tubers are wonderfully rich in flavor and nutrients; they deserve to be an everyday vegetable, not just a holiday side dish.

Their fiber alone is enough to make sweet potatoes worth eating, since a diet rich in fiber is associated with a lower risk of all sorts of health problems, from heart attacks to constipation. Sweet potatoes also provide an enormous helping of vitamin A in the form of antioxidant beta-carotene, making it a top-flight weapon for fighting chronic diseases such as cancer and heart disease, as well as inflammation-related conditions such as asthma and rheumatoid arthritis. The sweet potato is also rich in vitamin C, which helps boost immunity and fight infections, and in potassium, which helps lower blood pressure.

# SWEET POTATO FRIES

1 **large sweet potato (about 8 ounces)**

1 **tablespoon olive oil**

¼ **teaspoon coarse salt**

¼ **teaspoon black pepper**

¼ **teaspoon ground red pepper**

**Honey or maple syrup (optional)**

**1** Preheat oven to 425°F. Peel sweet potato; cut lengthwise into long spears.

**2** Combine sweet potato, oil, salt, black pepper and red pepper in medium bowl; toss to coat. Arrange in single layer on large baking sheet.

**3** Bake 20 to 30 minutes or until sweet potato is lightly browned, turning halfway through baking time. Serve with honey, if desired.

*Makes 2 servings*

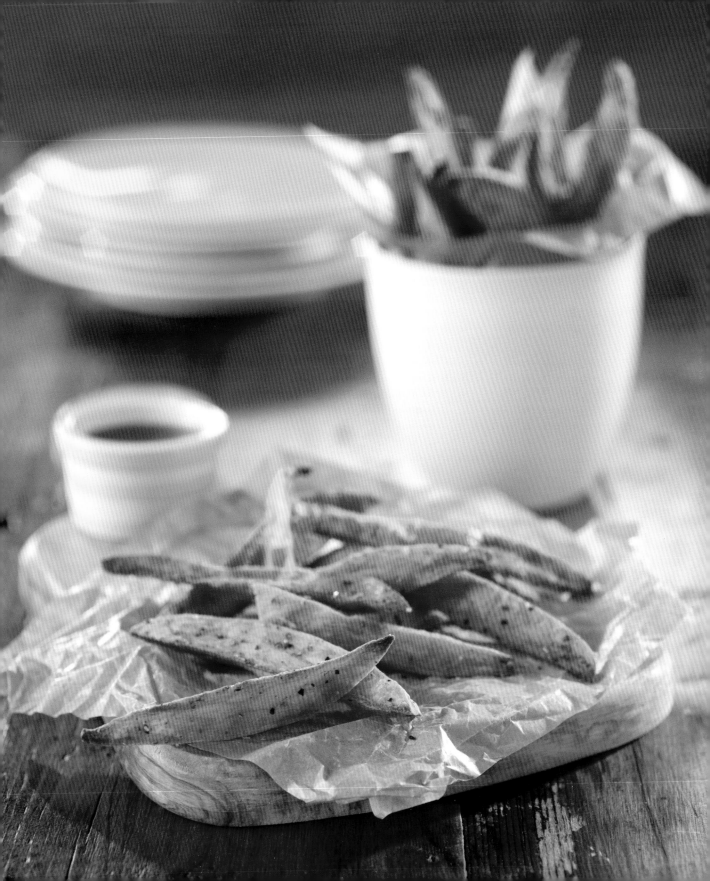

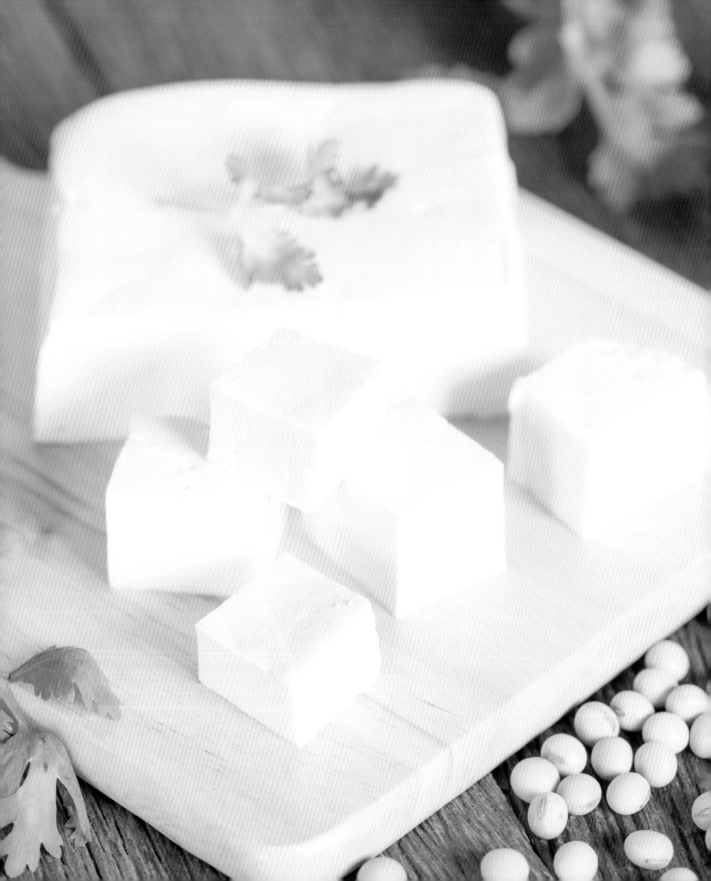

# TOFU

A nutritionally complete protein, tofu can be stir-fried, grilled, poached, baked or blended into sauces or smoothies. The mild, clean taste works well with a wide range of ingredients and flavors, from rich and hearty to hot and spicy.

Tofu contains all the amino acids we need from food; it also supplies beneficial amounts of iron, key to getting oxygen to our cells. Like other soy foods containing soy isoflavones and phytonutrients, tofu has been linked to less risk of heart disease and some cancers and relief of menopausal symptoms. And soy protein also appears to help lower levels of LDL cholesterol.

# VEGETARIAN RICE NOODLES

½ **cup soy sauce**

⅓ **cup sugar**

¼ **cup lime juice**

2 **fresh red Thai chiles** *or*
 **1 large jalapeño pepper,***
 **finely chopped**

8 **ounces thin rice noodles**
 **(rice vermicelli)**

¼ **cup vegetable oil**

8 **ounces firm tofu, drained**
 **and cut into triangles**

1 **jicama (8 ounces), peeled**
 **and chopped** *or* **1 can**
 **(8 ounces) sliced water**
 **chestnuts, drained**

2 **medium sweet potatoes**
 **(1 pound), peeled and cut**
 **into ¼-inch-thick slices**

2 **large leeks, cut into**
 **¼-inch-thick slices**

¼ **cup chopped unsalted**
 **dry-roasted peanuts**

2 **tablespoons chopped**
 **fresh mint**

2 **tablespoons chopped**
 **fresh cilantro**

*\*Chile peppers can sting and irritate
the skin, so wear rubber gloves when
handling peppers and do not touch
your eyes.*

**1** Combine soy sauce, sugar, lime juice and
chiles in small bowl; mix well.

**2** Place rice noodles in medium bowl. Cover
with hot water; let stand 15 minutes or until
soft. Drain well; cut into 3-inch lengths.

**3** Meanwhile, heat oil in large skillet over
medium-high heat. Add tofu; stir-fry
4 minutes per side or until golden brown.
Remove with slotted spatula to paper
towel-lined baking sheet.

**4** Add jicama to skillet; stir-fry 5 minutes or
until lightly browned. Remove to baking
sheet. Stir-fry sweet potatoes in batches
until tender and browned; remove to
baking sheet. Add leeks; stir-fry 1 minute;
remove to baking sheet.

**5** Stir soy sauce mixture; add to skillet. Heat
until sugar dissolves. Add noodles; toss
to coat. Gently stir in tofu, vegetables,
peanuts, mint and cilantro; cook until
heated through.

*Makes 4 servings*

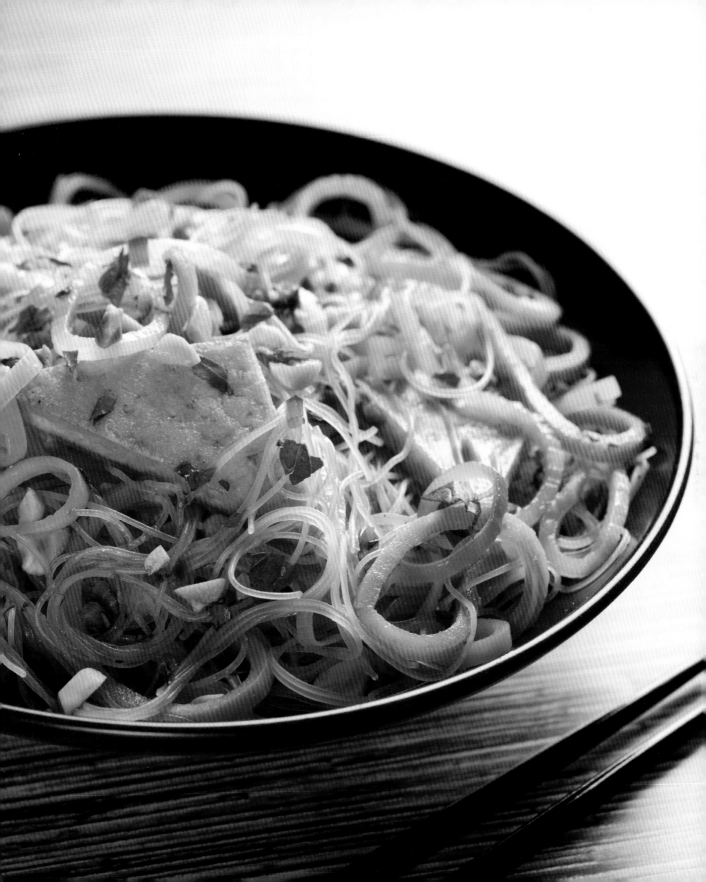

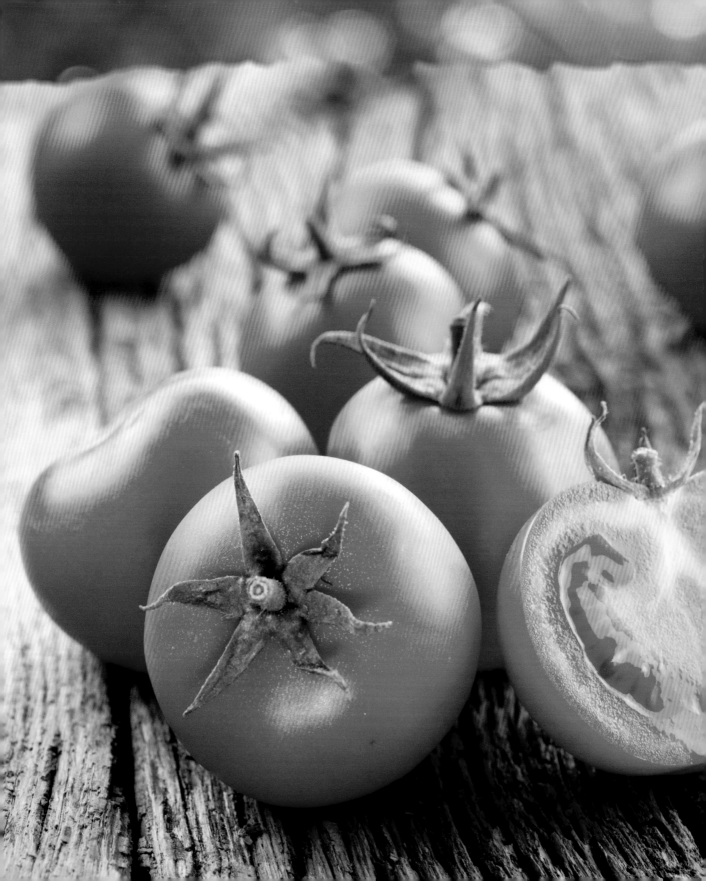

# TOMATOES

Although technically a fruit, tomatoes are one of the world's most popular vegetables. Raw or cooked, in sauces or salads, tomatoes add color, flavor and texture to every kind of dish.

Tomatoes are rich in lycopene, an antioxidant that gives the tomato its red color and may help reduce the risk of cardiovascular disease and prostate cancer. The vitamin C in tomatoes is an antioxidant that supports healthy immune function, while their beta-carotene and other carotenoids are powerful weapons against heart disease, cancer and other chronic ills. Tomatoes are also an important source of potassium, a mineral that is critical to heart, muscle and nerve functions.

# MARINATED TOMATO SALAD

1½ **cups white wine vinegar**

½ **teaspoon salt**

¼ **cup finely chopped shallots**

2 **tablespoons finely chopped chives**

2 **tablespoons lemon juice**

¼ **teaspoon white pepper**

2 **tablespoons extra virgin olive oil**

6 **plum tomatoes, quartered**

2 **large yellow tomatoes,\* cut horizontally into ½-inch-thick slices**

16 **red cherry tomatoes, halved**

**Sunflower sprouts (optional)**

*\*Substitute 10 plum tomatoes, quartered, for yellow tomatoes, if desired.*

1 Combine vinegar and salt in large bowl; stir until salt is completely dissolved. Add shallots, chives, lemon juice and pepper; mix well. Slowly whisk in oil until well blended.

2 Add tomatoes to marinade; toss to coat. Cover and let stand at room temperature 30 minutes or up to 2 hours before serving. Garnish with sunflower sprouts.

*Makes 8 servings*

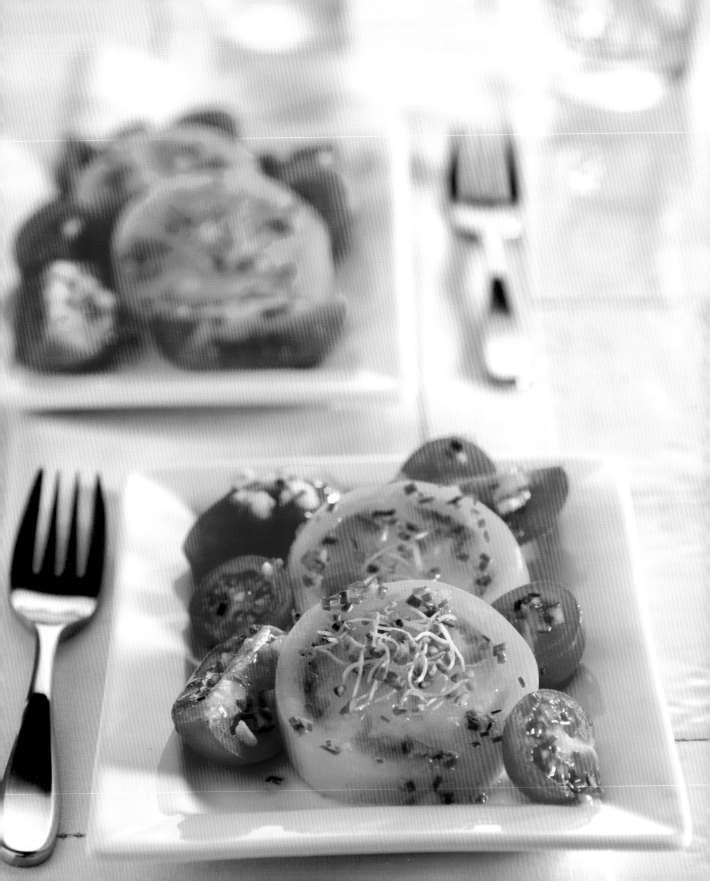

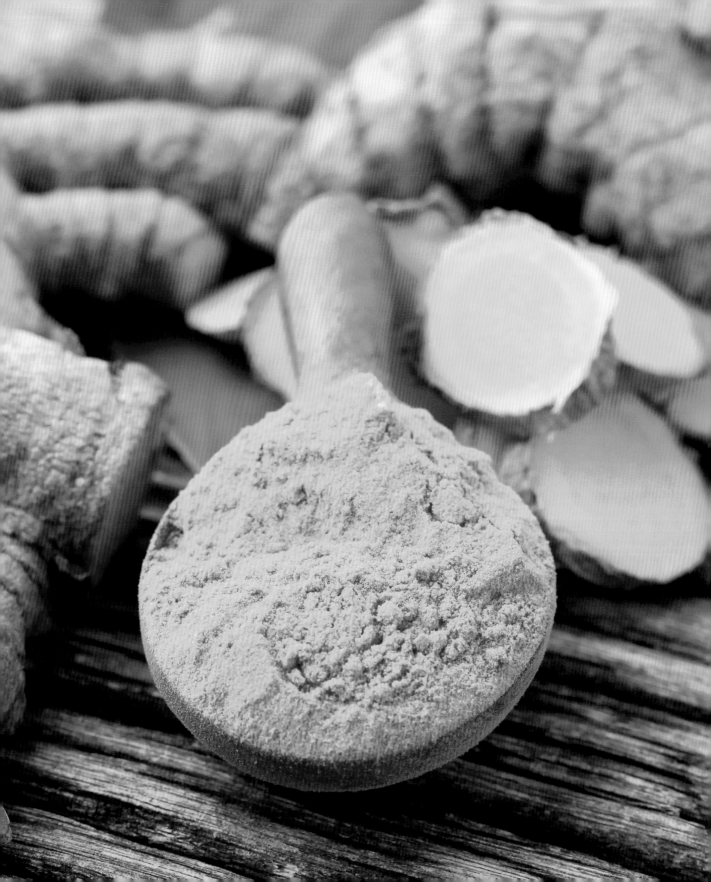

# TURMERIC

Known as "the golden spice," turmeric has been a staple in Southeast Asian and Middle Eastern cooking for thousands of years and is easily recognized by its bright yellow color.

The main active ingredient in turmeric, curcumin, is a strong antioxidant, helping to fight cancer-causing free radicals and boost the body's own antioxidant mechanisms. It also has potent anti-inflammatory properties, which may help treat gastrointestinal and menstrual issues (reducing irritation throughout the gut while contributing to healthy digestion), and it may assist in relieving pain and swelling in people with osteo and rheumatoid arthritis. Other possible benefits of turmeric include improving liver function and reducing levels of toxicity in the body, and some studies suggest that it may protect against some types of cancers.

# SPICY CHICKPEAS
## AND COUSCOUS

1 **can (about 14 ounces) vegetable broth**

1 **teaspoon ground coriander**

½ **teaspoon ground cardamom**

½ **teaspoon ground turmeric**

½ **teaspoon hot pepper sauce**

¼ **teaspoon salt**

⅛ **teaspoon ground cinnamon**

1 **cup matchstick-size carrots**

1 **can (about 15 ounces) chickpeas, rinsed and drained**

1 **cup frozen green peas**

1 **cup quick-cooking couscous**

2 **tablespoons chopped fresh mint or parsley**

**1** Combine broth, coriander, cardamom, turmeric, hot pepper sauce, salt and cinnamon in large saucepan; bring to a boil over high heat. Add carrots; cook over medium heat 5 minutes.

**2** Add chickpeas and green peas; return to a simmer. Cook 2 minutes.

**3** Stir in couscous. Remove from heat; cover and let stand 5 minutes or until liquid is absorbed. Sprinkle with mint.

*Makes 6 servings*

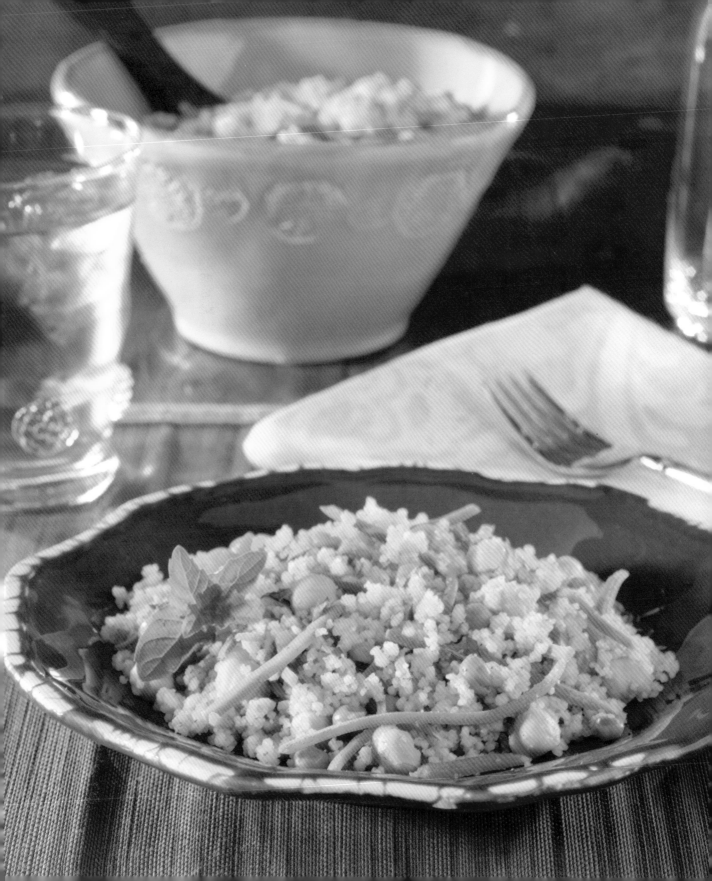

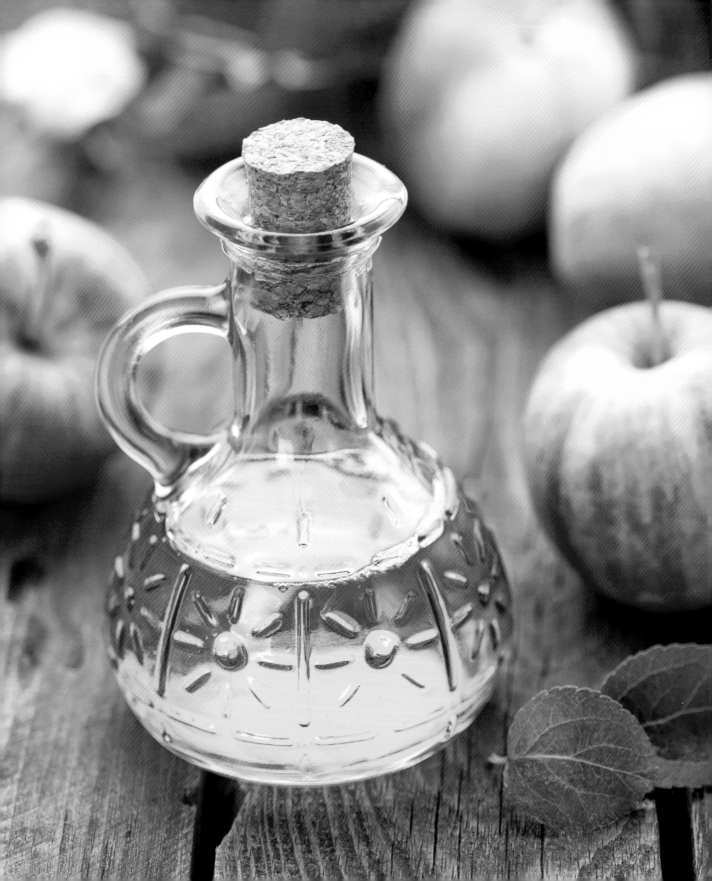

# VINEGAR

With its high acid content, drinking vinegar straight isn't recommended. But adding some vinegar to your diet can provide a wide range of potential benefits.

Vinegar increases the acidity in the stomach, which allows it to digest the food you've eaten and move it to the small intestine, thus reducing bloating. Vinegar can help your body absorb the nutrients in the food you eat, slow the rush of sugar to your bloodstream, and possibly minimize a blood sugar spike after a large intake of sugar or carbs. Some studies have suggested that vinegar may help regulate blood sugar and improve blood glucose levels. For those with diabetes or pre-diabetes, it may help improve insulin sensitivity. And despite its acidic nature, vinegar can help balance pH levels in the body with naturally occurring enzymes and probiotics which may lead to better bone health.

# SWEET AND SOUR RED CABBAGE

1 slice bacon, chopped

½ cup chopped sweet or yellow onion

4 cups thinly sliced red cabbage

1 unpeeled red apple, cut into ½-inch pieces

¼ cup cider vinegar

¼ cup honey

½ teaspoon celery salt

1 Cook bacon in large deep skillet over medium heat until crisp, stirring frequently. Drain on paper towel-lined plate.

2 Add onion to drippings in skillet; cook 5 minutes or until onion is softened, stirring occasionally.

3 Add cabbage, apple, vinegar, honey and celery salt to skillet; cook and stir 12 to 14 minutes or until cabbage is crisp-tender and liquid is reduced to a glaze.* Sprinkle with bacon.

*For more tender cabbage, cover and cook 15 minutes, then uncover and cook until liquid is reduced to a glaze.*

**Makes 4 servings**

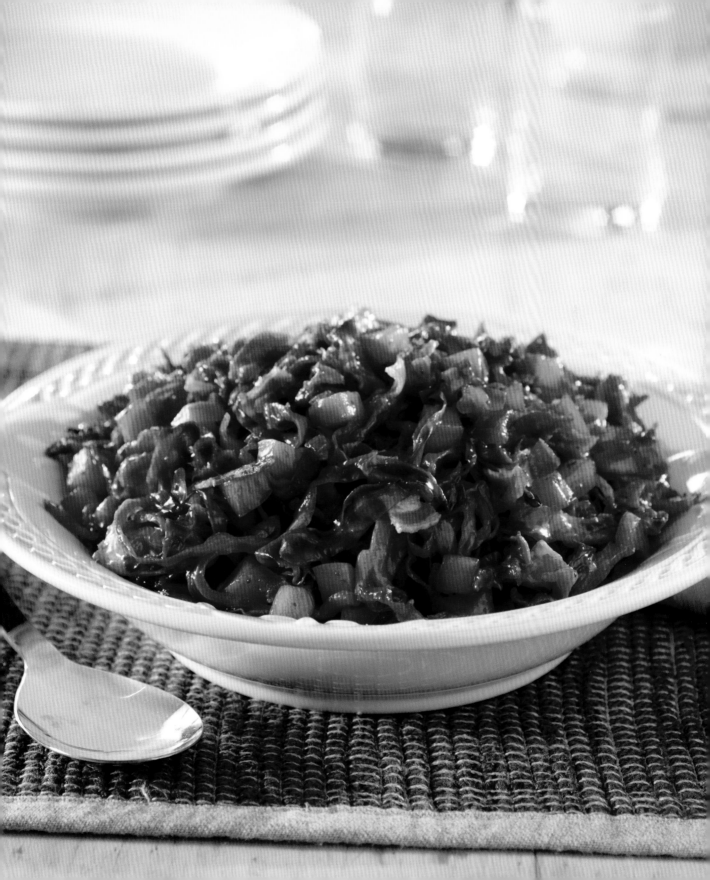

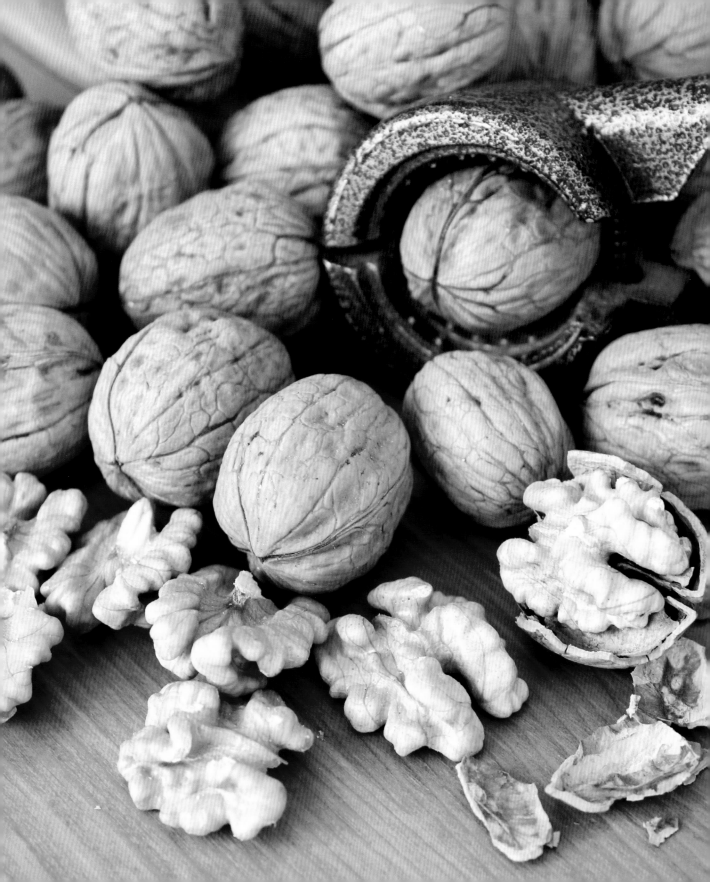

# WALNUTS

The ancient Romans called walnuts the food of the gods, and they do contain a wealth of nutritional benefits.

Compared to other nuts, walnuts provide the most alpha-linolenic acid, the plant-based source of omega-3 fats that helps prevent blood clotting, reduce inflammation and lower triglyceride levels in the blood. Other common nuts also trail far behind walnuts in the amount and quality of their antioxidants, which boost disease resistance and protect the body's cells from damage. Plus, walnuts supply protein and soluble fiber to help satisfy hunger, lower blood cholesterol and keep blood sugar in check.

# ROASTED VEGETABLE SALAD WITH CAPERS AND WALNUTS

1   pound small brussels sprouts, trimmed

1   pound unpeeled small Yukon Gold potatoes, cut into halves

½   teaspoon salt, divided

¼   teaspoon black pepper

¼   teaspoon dried rosemary

5   tablespoons olive oil, divided

1   red bell pepper, cut into bite-size pieces

¼   cup walnuts, coarsely chopped

2   tablespoons capers, drained

1½   tablespoons white wine vinegar

**1**   Preheat oven to 400°F.

**2**   Slash bottoms of brussels sprouts; place on large baking sheet. Add potatoes; sprinkle with ¼ teaspoon salt, black pepper and rosemary. Drizzle with 3 tablespoons oil; toss to coat. Roast 20 minutes.

**3**   Stir in bell pepper; roast 15 minutes or until tender. Transfer to large bowl; stir in walnuts and capers.

**4**   Whisk remaining 2 tablespoons oil, vinegar and remaining ¼ teaspoon salt in small bowl until blended. Pour over salad; toss to coat. Serve at room temperature.

*Makes 6 servings*

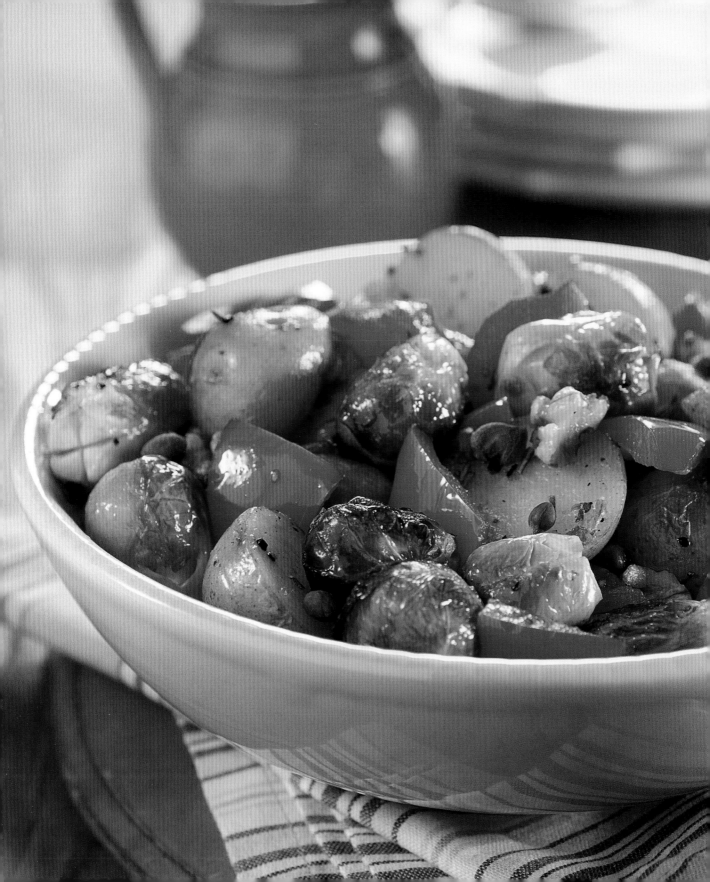

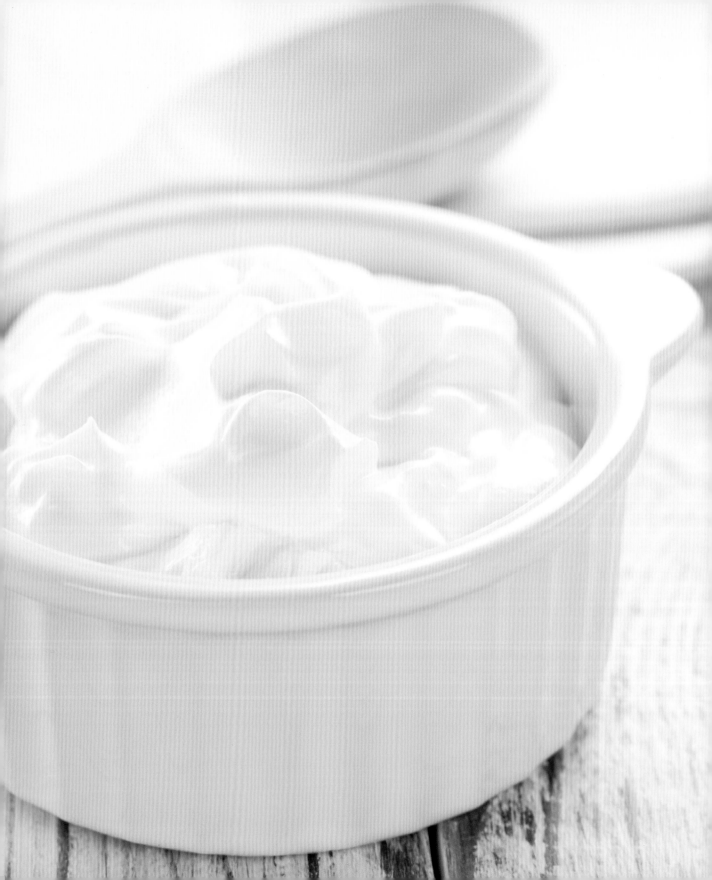

# YOGURT

Yogurt is a nutrient-rich source of protein that has the health benefits of milk and more.

Since it is made from milk, it offers as much bone-building calcium as milk but is digested more easily since it contains live active bacterial cultures. These active bacteria also improve your immune system, suppress the growth of harmful bacteria in the intestine and help lower LDL cholesterol. You can further enhance the benefits by selecting yogurt with added vitamin D. Research suggests yogurt with active cultures may help combat a variety of gastrointestinal problems—such as constipation, diarrhea, lactose intolerance, ulcer, inflammatory bowel disease and possibly colon cancer—by bolstering the body's immune response and rebalancing microorganisms naturally present in the gut.

# TANDOORI CHICKEN SANDWICHES WITH YOGURT SAUCE

4 **boneless skinless chicken breasts (about 1 pound)**

1 **tablespoon lemon juice**

¼ **cup plain yogurt**

2 **cloves garlic, minced**

1½ **teaspoons finely chopped fresh ginger**

¼ **teaspoon ground cardamom**

¼ **teaspoon ground red pepper**

**Yogurt Sauce (recipe follows)**

2 **whole wheat pita bread rounds**

½ **cup grated carrot**

½ **cup finely shredded red cabbage**

½ **cup finely chopped red bell pepper**

**1** Lightly score chicken breasts three or four times with sharp knife. Place in medium bowl; sprinkle with lemon juice and toss to coat.

**2** Combine yogurt, garlic, ginger, cardamom and ground red pepper in small bowl; mix well. Add to chicken; turn pieces to coat completely. Cover and refrigerate at least 1 hour or overnight.

**3** Remove chicken from refrigerator 15 minutes before cooking. Preheat broiler. Prepare Yogurt Sauce.

**4** Line broiler pan with foil. Arrange chicken on foil (do not let pieces touch) and brush with any remaining marinade.

**5** Broil 3 inches from heat 5 to 6 minutes per side or until chicken is no longer pink in center.

**6** Cut pita rounds in half crosswise; gently open. Place one chicken breast in each pita half with 2 tablespoons each of carrot, cabbage and bell pepper. Drizzle with Yogurt Sauce.

*Makes 4 servings*

**YOGURT SAUCE:** Combine ½ cup plain yogurt, 2 teaspoons minced red onion, 1 teaspoon minced fresh cilantro, ¼ teaspoon salt, ¼ teaspoon ground cumin and dash of ground red pepper in small bowl; mix well. Refrigerate until ready to serve.

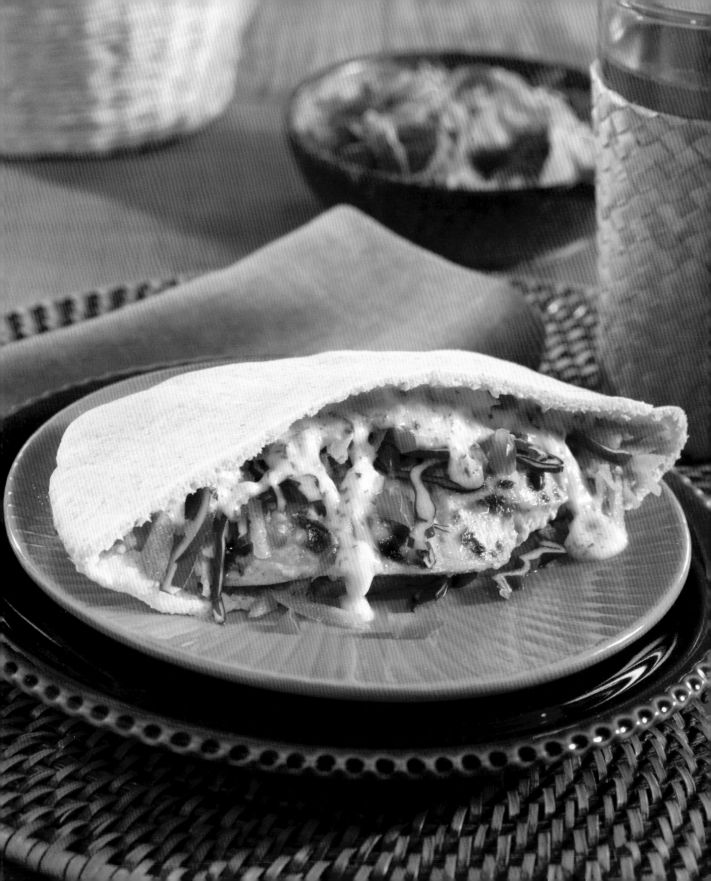

# INDEX

# METRIC CONVERSION CHART

## VOLUME MEASUREMENTS (dry)

1/8 teaspoon = 0.5 mL
1/4 teaspoon = 1 mL
1/2 teaspoon = 2 mL
3/4 teaspoon = 4 mL
1 teaspoon = 5 mL
1 tablespoon = 15 mL
2 tablespoons = 30 mL
1/4 cup = 60 mL
1/3 cup = 75 mL
1/2 cup = 125 mL
2/3 cup = 150 mL
3/4 cup = 175 mL
1 cup = 250 mL
2 cups = 1 pint = 500 mL
3 cups = 750 mL
4 cups = 1 quart = 1 L

## VOLUME MEASUREMENTS (fluid)

1 fluid ounce (2 tablespoons) = 30 mL
4 fluid ounces (1/2 cup) = 125 mL
8 fluid ounces (1 cup) = 250 mL
12 fluid ounces (1 1/2 cups) = 375 mL
16 fluid ounces (2 cups) = 500 mL

## WEIGHTS (mass)

1/2 ounce = 15 g
1 ounce = 30 g
3 ounces = 90 g
4 ounces = 120 g
8 ounces = 225 g
10 ounces = 285 g
12 ounces = 360 g
16 ounces = 1 pound = 450 g

## DIMENSIONS

1/16 inch = 2 mm
1/8 inch = 3 mm
1/4 inch = 6 mm
1/2 inch = 1.5 cm
3/4 inch = 2 cm
1 inch = 2.5 cm

## OVEN TEMPERATURES

250°F = 120°C
275°F = 140°C
300°F = 150°C
325°F = 160°C
350°F = 180°C
375°F = 190°C
400°F = 200°C
425°F = 220°C
450°F = 230°C

## BAKING PAN SIZES

| Utensil | Size in Inches/Quarts | Metric Volume | Size in Centimeters |
|---|---|---|---|
| Baking or Cake Pan (square or rectangular) | 8×8×2 | 2 L | 20×20×5 |
| | 9×9×2 | 2.5 L | 23×23×5 |
| | 12×8×2 | 3 L | 30×20×5 |
| | 13×9×2 | 3.5 L | 33×23×5 |
| Loaf Pan | 8×4×3 | 1.5 L | 20×10×7 |
| | 9×5×3 | 2 L | 23×13×7 |
| Round Layer Cake Pan | 8×1½ | 1.2 L | 20×4 |
| | 9×1½ | 1.5 L | 23×4 |
| Pie Plate | 8×1¼ | 750 mL | 20×3 |
| | 9×1¼ | 1 L | 23×3 |
| Baking Dish or Casserole | 1 quart | 1 L | — |
| | 1½ quart | 1.5 L | — |
| | 2 quart | 2 L | — |